KU-374-438

TABLE OF CONTENTS

THIRD EDITION

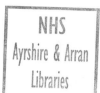

NURSING PROCESS

CONCEPTS AND APPLICATION

Australia • Brazil • Japan • Korea • Mexico • Singapore • Spain • United Kingdom • United States

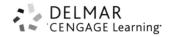

Nursing Process: Concepts and Application, International Edition
Wanda Walker Seaback

Vice President, Editorial: Dave Garza

Executive Editor: Stephen Helba

Associate Acquisitions Editor:
Delia K. Uherec

Managing Editor: Marah Bellegarde

Editorial Assistant: Jennifer Wheaton

Vice President, Marketing: Jennifer Baker

Marketing Director: Wendy E. Mapstone

Executive Marketing Manager:
Michele McTighe

Associate Marketing Manager:
Scott A. Chrysler

Production Director:
Wendy A. Troeger

Production Manager: Andrew Crouth

Design Direction, Production Management,
and Composition: PreMediaGlobal

Library of Congress Control Number: 2012934271

International Edition:

ISBN-13: 978-1-111-30825-4

ISBN-10: 1-111-30825-X

Cengage Learning International Offices

Asia
www.cengageasia.com
tel: (65) 6410 1200

Australia/New Zealand
www.cengage.com.au
tel: (61) 3 9685 4111

Brazil
www.cengage.com.br
tel: (55) 11 3665 9900

India
www.cengage.co.in
tel: (91) 11 4364 1111

Latin America
www.cengage.com.mx
tel: (52) 55 1500 6000

UK/Europe/Middle East/Africa
www.cengage.co.uk
tel: (44) 0 1264 332 424

**Represented in Canada by
Nelson Education, Ltd.**
tel: (416) 752 9100 / (800) 668 0671
www.nelson.com

Cengage Learning is a leading provider of customized learning solutions with office locations around the globe, including Singapore, the United Kingdom, Australia, Mexico, Brazil, and Japan. Locate your local office at:
www.cengage.com/global

For product information and free companion resources:
www.cengage.com/international
Visit your local office: **www.cengage.com/global**

Printed in the United States of America
1 2 3 4 5 6 7 16 15 14 13 12

To George, my husband. Thank you for your love, continued support over the years, and always believing in me.

PREFACE

Nursing Process: Concepts and Application was written with the educator and nursing student in mind. Most educators will agree that nursing process is one of the most important concepts to be taught in fundamental nursing. Most theories presented in nursing textbooks are based on the nursing process steps: assessment, problem identification/diagnosis, planning and outcome identification, implementation, and evaluation. National licensing examination questions are formatted and written utilizing the nursing process.

The student textbook is written to correspond with the educator's PowerPoint presentation/lecture material (available through Delmar Cengage Learning). Numerous learning activities and key points are included throughout each chapter, thus promoting interactive learning and stimulating questions and in-class discussion. Activities are included that assist student in understanding the presented concepts and theory and for practical application of these concepts. The information is presented in a clear, uncluttered approach emphasizing application.

Key Features:

- Presents the nursing process in an easy-to-understand, step-by-step format.
- Student Practice activities promote application of the concept behind each step.
- Student Practice activities build upon one another, increasing in complexity to promote understanding, critical thinking, and practical application of each step of the nursing process.
- Numerous examples and cases allow students to apply their knowledge as they progress through the text.
- Nursing Tips provide students with practical hints that can be used in the learning and working environment.

WHAT'S NEW IN THE THIRD EDITION?

Sample chapters of the first draft were selected and sent for review by nurse educators in colleges of nursing throughout the United States. Reviewers were faculty in licensed vocational/practical nursing programs, associate degree and baccalaureate programs. Those nursing professionals were asked specific questions, such as, what was liked about the sample, what was not liked, and what would improve the textbook. These comments were shared with the author and have been used to guide the revisions and additions in the third edition, which include the following:

- Additional theory, student reflections, and graphics have been included. Chapter 1 provides an overview of theoretical concepts and foundation information. Chapters 2 through 6 discuss each step of the nursing process, introducing key terms, examples, points to remember, and learning activities. Chapter 7 helps the student put it all together. A clinical case study is presented and the author takes the student through each step.

Also included in the third edition is a chapter introducing Concept Mapping. Data presented in the final Chapter 7 scenario is utilized to build the concept map.
- A new chapter, Chapter 8, introduces Concept Mapping principles as well as provides application exercises for student.
- NANDA diagnoses have been updated throughout.
- New feature, Reflections, is designed to provide application of concepts within the learning process.
- Nursing Tips have been updated to provide targeted application in the learning and working environment.

INSTRUCTOR RESOURCES

Available via an instructor account on cengage.com:
- Updated PowerPoint slides designed to enhance your class presentation.
- Suggested answers to the student activities and case studies.
- Updated Test Bank with NCLEX style questions.

Instructors: If you do not currently have a Cengage.com Instructor Account, please visit Cengage.com or contact your sales representative to sign up!

CONCEPT

In developing this textbook, I desired a work that could be adapted to all levels of nursing education, beginning with vocational/practical, applied science/associate degree nursing, and then broadening concepts and theory to embrace baccalaureate nursing. I believed it was important to present essential material students must learn and understand in order to apply the nursing process in clinical practice. All beginning nursing students must have a strong foundation and solid understanding of fundamental concepts.

I was motivated to provide important basic information to guide the reader, step-by-step, so that each student could understand and apply the nursing process concepts. Since its initial development in 1996, a great deal of the content has been rewritten and revised for clarity and effectiveness to benefit students' understanding. I am pleased to find that nursing students, through the use of this text, are able to understand the concepts and demonstrate the ability to apply this knowledge in clinical practice. *Nursing Process: Concepts and Application* is the culmination of this endeavor.

The author invites students and nursing professors to send comments or recommendations via e-mail. Many of your observations and annotations have been influential in the revisions of this manuscript.

Email: **wseaback@tamhsc.edu**

REVIEWERS

The author would like to thank the following reviewers for their valuable input:

Kim Baily, RN, MSN, PhD
Director of Nursing
El Camino College
Torrance, California

Patty Hawley, MSE
Allied Health Instructor
Ferris State University
Big Rapids, Michigan

Sheri Hawley, BSN
Practical Nursing Instructor
College of Southern Idaho
Twin Falls, Idaho

Cheryl Martin, PhD, RNC-OB, WHNP-BC, CNE
Associate Professor of Nursing
University of Indianapolis
Indianapolis, Indiana

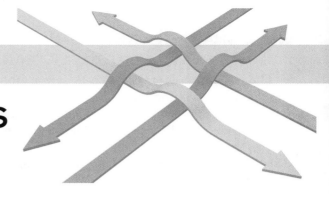

CHAPTER 1

NURSING PROCESS AND PROVIDING CARE

KEY TERMS

assessment
care plan
client centered
collaboration
critical thinking
decision making
diagnosis

evaluation
expected outcome
goal
implementation
The Joint Commission
medical diagnosis
NANDA

nursing diagnosis
nursing intervention
nursing process
prioritize
problem solving

The nursing process is a step-by-step method of providing care to clients. While progressing through each step, the nurse uses a variety of skills that are purposeful and promote a systematic, orderly thought process. The nursing process consists of five steps—assessment, diagnosis, planning and outcome identification, implementation, and evaluation.

This chapter provides a brief historical time line of the evolution of the nursing process (see Table 1:1), its outstanding characteristics, and an overview of each step. Chapter topics include discussion of the theoretical basis of the nursing process, the importance and necessity of critical thinking throughout all steps of the process, and the relationship among problem solving, decision making, and the nursing process.

John T., the nurse, receives a shift report less than an hour ago on his assigned group of patients. As he organizes his notes, preparing for the day, the nursing assistant reports an extremely elevated blood pressure (210/108 mm Hg) for Mrs. Simpson in room 214-B.

Clinical situations, such as the scenario above, are likely to occur in most health care institutions. If *you* are the nurse, what will you do next? What is the priority for care? What questions will you ask? What actions will you take?

Understanding and applying concepts of the nursing process will help the nurse identify priorities, plan, provide health care, and evaluate patient progress. What is the *nursing process*?

Read on for the definition of the nursing process and examples of application!

NURSING PROCESS

The nursing process is defined as an organized, systematic method of planning and providing individualized care to clients. The nursing process is a tool promoting organization and utilization of the steps to achieve desired outcomes. The steps of the nursing process build upon each other, overlapping previous and subsequent steps. The nursing process may be used with clients throughout their life span and in any setting where care is provided to clients.

Unique Characteristics of the Nursing Process

The nursing process is a problem-solving and decision-making method that is scientifically, as well as philosophically, based. The nurse uses learned knowledge and understanding of the human body to identify actual or potential health problems resulting from physical or psychological diseases or disorders. Knowledge and understanding of fundamental philosophical views, such as Maslow's hierarchy of human needs (Figure 1:1), are essential to the practice of nursing and aid in identifying the expected response to illness or the client's sense of wellness.

The nursing process is cyclic, ongoing, and dynamic. Using an orderly, step-by-step process, the client is evaluated, data are collected and analyzed, and a plan is formulated and set into motion. Client progress and response to treatment are continuously monitored and evaluated. The care plan is revised according to the changing needs of the client.

The nursing process is a method used to organize nursing activities. The ultimate goal is to promote and restore client wellness or to maintain the client's present state of health or sense of wellness.

TABLE 1:1 Timeline: Evolution of the Nursing Process

pre-1955	Before the nursing process evolved, the nurse provided care based on medical orders written by physicians. Care was initiated based on the caregiver's instinct to nurture. There were no clearly identifiable boundaries defined for nursing practice.
1955	The term *nursing process* was coined by Lydia Hall.
Late 1950s–early 1960s	Dorothy Johnson (1959), Ida Orlando (1961), and Ernestine Wiedenbach (1963) introduced a three-step nursing process model.
1966	Virginia Henderson identified the nursing process model as the same steps used in the scientific method: observing, measuring, gathering data, and analyzing the findings.
1967	A four-step model was proposed: assessment, planning, intervention, and evaluation.
1973	The use of the nursing process in clinical practice continued to gain additional accuracy and recognition when the American Nurses Association (ANA) published *Standards of Clinical Nursing Practice* (Table 1:2).
	Publication of Standards gave further legitimacy to the five phases or steps of the nursing process. Nursing educators and clinicians began to use the five-step nursing process model on a regular basis. National conferences were initiated in 1973, resulting in the beginning of the classification of nursing diagnoses. North American Nursing Diagnosis Association (NANDA) conferences have been held every 2 years since then for the purpose of identification, clarification, and refinement of nursing diagnoses.
1980	ANA published a social policy statement, which provided guidelines (standards) for individual professional nurses to follow in practice.
1982	National Council Licensure Examination (NCLEX) was revised to include the nursing process concepts as a basis for organization.
1984	Joint Commission on Accreditation of Healthcare Organizations (JCAHO) launched requirements for accredited hospitals to use the nursing process as a means of documenting all phases of client care. Note: JCAHO is now known as the Joint Commission.
Current	The nursing process is a five-step process: assessment, diagnosis, planning, implementation, and evaluation.

TABLE 1:2 Scope and Standards of Practice

Standard 1	*Assessment* Collects data
Standard 2	*Diagnosis* Analyzes data
Standard 3	*Outcomes Identification* Individualizes expected outcomes for client
Standard 4	*Planning* Develops plan of care
Standard 5	*Implementation* Implements interventions in plan of care
Standard 6	*Evaluation* Determines client progress toward outcome achievement

From American Nurses Association (2010). *Nursing: Scope and standards of practice.* 2nd Edition, Washington, DC: Author.

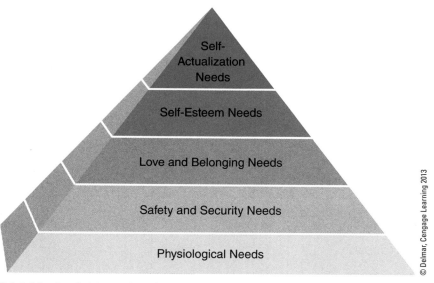

© Delmar, Cengage Learning 2013

FIGURE 1:1 Maslow's hierarchy of needs. All human beings have common basic needs that must be met to some degree before higher-level needs are met.

TABLE 1:3 Comparing Nursing and Nonnursing Models

Nursing Models	Nonnursing Models
• Functional health patterns • Human response pattern • Theory of self-care	• Body systems model • Hierarchy of needs

Assessment models provide a systematic method for organizing data. Both nursing and nonnursing models (e.g., medical, psychology) are utilized (see Table 1:3).

The nursing process is recognized to be highly effective in promoting quality of care. A client entering the health care continuum receives a thorough initial assessment. The needs of the client are identified. A care plan (documentation of the first, second, and third steps of the nursing process) is developed and communicated to other health care professionals, so care is coordinated and ongoing. The client is continuously monitored for changing needs, and the plan is evaluated for accuracy. Assessment and evaluation, which are constant, play key roles in realizing client needs, strengths, and response to treatment. Health care professionals review, revise, and validate the care plan, enhancing and promoting quality of care.

The nursing process serves as a guide, ensuring deliberate steps are taken that help avoid omissions and premature conclusions. It provides a framework for which nurses use knowledge and skill to express human caring and to help clients meet their needs.

The nursing process is client centered, meaning care is focused on the client. The nurse organizes the care plan according to client problems, strengths, or both. The client is encouraged to be an active participant in the nursing process, communicating needs and concerns and validating collected data. This gives the client a sense of control over his or her care.

Throughout the nursing process, the nurse utilizes interpersonal, technical, and intellectual skills.

- Interpersonal skills include communicating, listening, conveying interest and compassion, and sharing knowledge and information. The use of interpersonal skills aids in promoting trust.
- Technical skills deal with operation of equipment and performance of procedures.
- Intellectual skills involve cognitive measures, such as analyzing, problem solving, critical thinking, and making judgments.

The nursing process promotes collaboration (communication with other disciplines to solve problems). As the client enters the health care system, individual professional responsibilities of the health care providers begin. Ongoing assessment of the client and response to care are monitored and recorded as physician orders and nursing interventions are carried out. Nursing professionals communicate necessary data through means of verbal reports and written documentation. Collaboration with the physician, nursing professionals, and other disciplines is often necessary to coordinate care and promote health.

The nursing process is universally applicable. It is appropriate to institute and apply the nursing process with clients of any age. The nursing process may be incorporated at any point on the wellness–illness continuum in a variety of health-related settings, including schools, hospitals, home health care facilities, and clinics and across specialties in hospital or acute care settings, including intensive care, pediatrics, labor and delivery, medical surgical units, and so on.

Use of the nursing process is beneficial to both the client and nurse. Examples of benefits include the following:

- Promotes improved quality and continuity of care
- Promotes and encourages client participation
- Delivery of care and problem solving are organized, continuous, and systematic
- Time and resources are utilized more efficiently
- Delivery of care, meeting expectations of both the health care consumer and standards of the nursing profession
- Holds all nurses accountable and responsible for assessment, diagnosis, planning, implementation, and evaluation of client care

Each step of the nursing process is specific, in sequence, and interrelated.

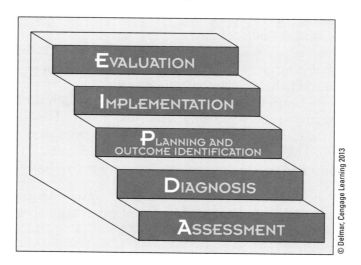

© Delmar, Cengage Learning 2013

Step 1: Assessment

Assessment provides significant information, assembled to form the client database. This phase involves several steps:

1. Data collection: through interviews, conversations, and performing physical assessment. A variety of sources may be utilized for the purpose of data collection, i.e., the client, family, significant other, and review of diagnostic examinations, laboratory results, and the client's chart.
2. Verification: validating accuracy of data will help prevent omissions, misunderstanding, and incorrect inferences.
3. Organization: categorizing or identifying patterns in data

4. Interpretation: formulating initial ideas or impressions
5. Documentation: recording or reporting data

Step 2: Diagnosis

Diagnosis is the classification of a disease, condition, or human response based upon scientific evaluation of signs and symptoms, patient history, and diagnostic studies. Diagnosis involves analysis of collected data. After analysis, a list of nursing diagnoses or labels describing client problems or strengths is formulated. The nurse uses critical-thinking and decision-making skills in developing nursing diagnoses, a process facilitated by asking questions such as:

• What actual problems, if any, were identified during the assessment step?
• What are the possible causes of the problems?
• Is the client at risk for developing other problems; if so, what are the factors involved?
• Did the client indicate a desire to function at a higher level of wellness in a particular area?
• What are the client's strengths?
• What additional data might be needed to answer these questions?
• What are possible sources of data collection?
• Are there any identified problems that should be treated in collaboration with the physician?
• What data are pertinent to collect before contacting the physician?

Clients receive both medical and nursing diagnoses. *Nursing diagnoses* should not be confused with *medical diagnoses*. Table 1:4 compares medical and nursing diagnoses.

Medical diagnoses are determined by the physician or nurse practitioner indicating a disease or disorder identified or to be ruled out, e.g., pneumonia, renal failure, sepsis, or diabetes mellitus. Nursing diagnoses are problems identified and determined by the professional nurse. So, *what makes the nursing diagnosis different?*

According to the NANDA, a nursing diagnosis is a clinical judgment about individual, family, or community responses to actual or potential health problems or life processes. In 1980, the ANA defined nursing process as the diagnosis and treatment of human responses to actual or potential health problems of disease and medical treatment.

So, what's the difference?

MD: "This client has pneumonia."

Nurse: "This client is experiencing ineffective breathing pattern."

© Delmar, Cengage Learning 2013

TABLE 1:4 Comparison of Medical Diagnoses and Nursing Diagnoses

Medical Diagnoses	Nursing Diagnoses
• Determined by the provider • Indicate a disease or disorder identified or to be ruled out • Remain constant until the client recovers from disease or illness	• Determined by nurses • Indicate the client's response to illness, disease, or present state of health • May change as the client responds to medical treatment, therapies, and nursing interventions
Examples:	**Examples:**
• Pneumonia • COPD exacerbation • Prostatitis • Acute renal failure	• Impaired gas exchange • Ineffective breathing pattern • Altered urinary elimination • Risk for impaired skin integrity

The preceding statement means nurses are *not* responsible for diagnosing and ordering treatment for disorders such as cancer. Professional nurses diagnose and treat the client's response to cancer, such as inadequate nutrition, nausea, altered self-esteem, anxiety, and pain.

After data are analyzed and problems, risks, and strengths identified, a list of nursing diagnoses is formulated and then presented to the client for confirmation. If the client is unable to participate, family members may be able to assist in confirmation. Finally, the list of nursing diagnoses is recorded and the remainder of the client's care plan completed.

During the nursing process, client is continuously reassessed (Figure 1:2). Data are collected and documented during this process. As physician-prescribed treatments and nurse-prescribed interventions are carried out, the client demonstrates responses to the care provided. Response to treatment may involve improvement of health or the client's condition may worsen. Nursing diagnoses included in the care plan reflect the changing needs of the client.

Step 3: Planning and Outcome Identification

Planning and outcome identification involves formulating and documenting the care plan. This phase of the nursing process organizes the proposed course of action for resolution of actual problems and prevention of risk problems. This task involves several steps:

1. Prioritizing nursing diagnoses
2. Identifying short- and long-term goals and expected outcomes
3. Determining nursing interventions that will aid in resolution or prevention of each problem

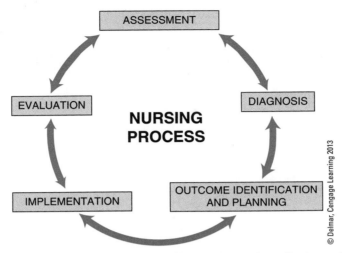

FIGURE 1:2 The nursing process is a method used to determine client needs. Assessment of the client and evaluation of the client and care plan are continuous. The nurse uses critical thinking, problem solving, and decision making throughout this process.

Prioritizing problems means to decide which nursing diagnoses are most important and require attention first. Problems involving life-threatening situations are given the highest priority. An in-depth discussion of prioritizing problems can be found in Chapter 4.

The absolute goal for any client is to achieve or maintain the greatest level of wellness possible. Goals are client centered, which means they focus on *behavior* of the client. Goals are broad statements describing the intended or desired change in the client's condition. An expected outcome is a particular expectation involving steps leading to the fulfillment of a goal and, therefore, resolution of the cause of a problem. Goals and expected outcomes are used to evaluate the effectiveness of nursing interventions and the care plan.

Nursing interventions are activities executed to enable accomplishment of goals. They are nursing actions planned and implemented with problem resolution in mind.

Step 4: Implementation

Implementation involves execution of the nursing care plan. As planned interventions are performed, the nurse must continue to assess the client's condition before, during, and after each intervention is carried out. Reporting and documentation of collected data are important. Both positive and negative responses are reported and documented. Negative responses to treatment may require additional intervention. Chapter 5 provides an in-depth discussion of implementation. Implementation includes:

1. Activating the plan of care
2. Carrying out planned interventions
3. Continued assessment as interventions are carried out
4. Recording and documenting care provided, interventions carried out, and client responses

TABLE 1:5 Questions to Ask during Evaluation

- Are the interventions working?
- Is the current care plan helping the client make progress toward the goal?
- Has the client's status changed in any way? If so, is the plan still valid?
- Was the goal met or partially met?
- Was the goal realistic?
- Is there more that the health care team can do?
- Was the time frame too optimistic?
- Are goals and nursing interventions appropriate for the client?

Step 5: Evaluation

During evaluation (careful consideration of results), the nurse determines if client goals were met, partially met, or not met. If the goal has been met, the nurse must decide if or when nursing activities will cease. This decision will depend on the client's status. Can the client maintain the present level of wellness? If the goal has been partially met or not met, the nurse reactivates each step of the nursing process. Data must be collected to determine why the goal was not achieved and what modifications to the care plan are necessary. Refer to Table 1:5 for sample questions nurses ask to evaluate client care.

COGNITIVE SKILLS

When a client enters the health care system, nurses are involved in decision making. Care is planned for the client based on facts continuously collected and analyzed throughout the nursing process. Skills vital to this process include critical thinking, problem solving, and decision making.

Nursing Tip

Critical thinkers ask questions, seek understanding of evidence, and identify and evaluate alternatives.

Critical Thinking

Critical thinking is a purposeful thought process incorporating various strategies in search of the meaning of data. Deliberate questions are asked in order to validate and evaluate evidence. Critical thinkers seek out explanations for what is happening. Examples of questions critical thinkers ask are found in Table 1:6.

Problem Solving

The nursing process is a problem-solving method. However, there is a difference between this method and the method used in solving daily problems. In both

TABLE 1:6 Questions Critical Thinkers May Ask

Assessment	Have any data been omitted? Are there any data to be verified or validated that otherwise would lead to possible inaccuracies?
Diagnosis	What meaning is attached to collected data? What else could this mean? When clustering data, is there a pattern indicating specific problems? Is the client demonstrating signs or symptoms indicating he or she is at risk of developing future problems? Do the nursing diagnosis label and etiology accurately describe the problem? Did the client have adequate input into problem identification?
Planning and Outcome Identification	What are priority problems? Why are these problems priorities? What are the goals for the client? Are these goals realistic? What else might be accomplished? What interventions can assist the client in goal attainment? Is collaboration with other medical or health-related sources beneficial at this time? What other resources could benefit the client? Are planned interventions appropriate for the client, nurse, and facility?
Implementation	Has the client's condition changed since the last interaction? What is the client's current status? What interventions should be carried out first? Is the client demonstrating improvement in health status? Did the executed intervention result in the expected response? Why did the client respond in that manner?
Evaluation	Is the client progressing toward goal attainment? Are goals being met or only partially met? Is there more that can be done to alter the situation? Can the care plan be revised to be more effective? Was information accurate when initial data were collected? Was assessment thorough? Was each additional step of the nursing process followed through appropriately? Should additional data be collected? How can the plan be revised to best suit the client's needs?

methods, information is gathered, problems are identified, specific problems are labeled, a plan is developed for solving the problem, the plan is put into action, and then the results are evaluated. However, in solving daily problems, plans are frequently based on incomplete data and sometimes on presumptions. This type of problem solving is more linear compared with the cyclic and ongoing nature of the nursing process. Nurses using the nursing process method of problem solving actively engage in taking deliberate steps and use critical thought to identify and solve problems.

Nursing Tip

Establishing priorities is the first element of planning. Examine the nursing diagnoses and rank them in order of importance (physiological and psychological).

Decision Making

Decision making, a skill used throughout the nursing process, is based on systematic and scientifically based theories. Appropriate decision making and problem solving result from the nurse's ability to think critically, using perceptual and intellectual skills. This results in accurate problem identification, generating a reflective care plan, and determining appropriate nursing interventions to aid in problem resolution. Interventions for each nursing diagnosis are selected based on scientific rationale, or *why* the intervention will work. An in-depth discussion of scientific rationales can be found in Chapter 4, "Planning."

KEY CONCEPTS

- The nursing process is an organized, continuous, systematic method of planning, providing care, and problem solving. It is cyclic, ongoing, and dynamic.
- When a client enters the health care system, the nursing process begins. Use of the nursing process improves quality of care provided and promotes continuity of care.
- The nursing process consists of five interrelated steps: assessment, diagnosis, planning and outcome identification, implementation, and evaluation.
- Data collection utilizes a variety of sources and tools (*assessment*). Efforts are instituted to prevent omission or collection of inaccurate data.
- Data are organized and analyzed. Problems, potential problems, and strengths are identified and labeled (*diagnosis*).
- During the planning and outcome identification step, nursing diagnoses are prioritized. The professional nurse makes decisions on an appropriate course of action. The plan focuses on the client.
- Interventions are carried out (*implementation*).
- *Evaluation* of the plan and reassessment of the client are ongoing and continuous. The care plan is revised and updated when the client's needs change in response to medical treatment, therapies, and nursing interventions.
- *Care plan* revision may be necessary when the goal of treatment is partially met or not met.
- The care plan is developed, recorded, and placed in the client's chart and then communicated to other health care team members. This promotes ongoing continuity of care. The plan is reviewed for accuracy according to the policy of the facility and revised when needed.
- Nurses use perceptual and intellectual skills such as critical thinking, problem solving, and decision making.

APPLICATION EXAMPLE 1: PROBLEM SOLVING

Rachel Hernandez, a nurse for several years, was getting ready for a busy week. She was to drop her daughter, Marie, off at school before reporting for her shift at the local hospital. Marie had not responded when she was called for breakfast.

Step 1: Assessment

Ms. Hernandez was concerned and began to investigate the situation. As she approached Marie, Marie's face looked flushed, and she complained of fatigue. When Ms. Hernandez got closer, she could see a red, raised rash all over Marie's face and arms. Marie began scratching and reported she itched. Ms. Hernandez assessed for additional signs and symptoms. Marie's oral temperature was 98.8°F, and the glands in her neck were slightly swollen. Numerous questions went through Ms. Hernandez's mind as she performed a physical assessment and asked important questions. Marie was adamant that she was not going to school looking like this!

Step 2: Diagnosis

Ms. Hernandez was unsure of Marie's medical diagnosis; however, she was able to identify two distinct problematic responses resulting from Marie's condition. The responses were labeled using approved NANDA nursing diagnoses:

Impaired Skin Integrity. Related to nurse: presence of unknown infectious process; as evidenced by (AEB): pruritus, erythematous (red), raised rash on face and arms.

Step 3: Planning

- Ms. Hernandez thought about the preceding problems and what could be done. During the planning phase, questions are asked relating to problem solving. Is collaboration with other experts necessary or warranted? What independent activities can be done that are within her scope of practice and knowledge? What outcome can and should be achieved? What steps should be taken to resolve the situation?
- Impaired skin integrity, the primary goal or outcome is for Marie to demonstrate evidence of timely healing of the skin lesions without complications and within a reasonable amount of time, such as over the next 72 hours.
- Next in planning is to develop a plan of action and determine priorities.

  1. Contact Marie's school to report that she will be absent for the day.
  2. Contact the family physician for an afternoon appointment.
  3. Stress not to scratch the lesions and to keep the area clean and dry.
  4. Provide instructions for taking Tylenol for an elevated temperature if needed.

Step 4: Implementation

- Continue to assess Marie as interventions are executed. Carry out and perform the planned interventions.

Step 5: Evaluation

- Evaluation involves asking questions such as: Did the plan work? Was the goal achieved? At the end of 72 hours, do the lesions appear to be healing? Have other problems been identified? Are there revisions to make in the care plan to make it more effective?

When Ms. Hernandez returned home from work, she continued her assessment and evaluation. Marie's body temperature had continued to rise to 102.2°F, and she began to vomit. This must be added to the problem list. What physiological effect could this have on the body? If long lasting, it could affect Marie's comfort, nutrition, and fluid status. The appropriate nursing diagnoses for these risk problems are as follows: *Risk for Altered Nutrition: Less Than Body Requirements* and *Risk for Fluid Volume Deficit*. The term *risk* is used because Marie could potentially develop the problematic responses (altered nutrition and fluid volume deficit) to her illness, although they have not yet occurred.

STUDENT PRACTICE: PROBLEM SOLVING USING THE NURSING PROCESS

Instructions

Read the scenario below and provide answers to the following:

a. List all problem(s).
b. From the problem list, identify one priority nursing diagnosis.
c. Locate and write the definition of the nursing diagnosis.
d. What are *related to* and *as evidenced by* criteria?

1. Terrence Bennet, 8 years old, was brought into the clinic by his grandmother. He presented with multiple lesions on his face and extremities that appeared to be erythematous, ulcerated, and moist with honey-colored crusts. Terrence reported that the lesions itched.

   a. _____

   _____

   b. _____

   _____

c. _____

_____

_____

d. _____

_____

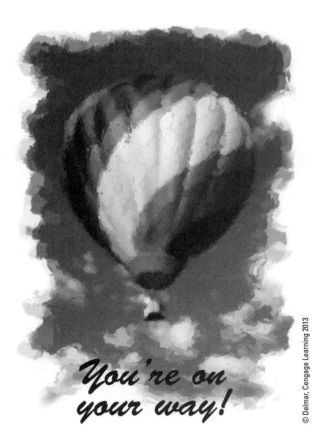

You're on your way!

2. Jay Mullins, 30 years old, was seen in the emergency clinic after sustaining an injury while playing football. He states he heard a "pop" when he was tackled and is now unable to support weight on his right ankle. He is experiencing pain rated as "8" on a scale of 0 to 10. His ankle has severe ecchymosis (bruising) and a large amount of tissue swelling around the fibula.

a. _____

_____

b. _____

_____

c. _____

_____

d. _____

_____

3. Martha Jacob, an 84-year-old woman, was seen in her primary care practitioner's office for a check-up 2 weeks after falling and sustaining a hip injury. She was treated at the time of her injury and released with no broken bones. She was to rest and take one Vicodin every 4 to 6 hours as needed for pain. Although Ms. Jacob reports the pain is somewhat better, her daughter expresses concern that her mother is not eating or drinking fluids well and her stools are hard and infrequent.

a. _____

_____

b. _____

_____

c. _____

_____

d. _____

_____

4. Charlotte Maxwell, 66 years old, is waiting to see her primary care physician. She is experiencing the following symptoms: discomfort when she urinates (dysuria) and a sense of urgency. Also, she is urinating more frequently but is voiding only small amounts of urine. Her symptoms have lasted for more than 1 week and are worsening.

a. _____

_____

b. _____

_____

c. _____

_____

d. _____

_____

CHAPTER 2

ASSESSMENT

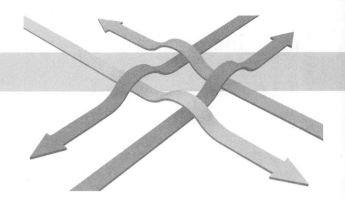

STANDARD 1: ASSESSMENT

Data collection

OBJECTIVES

Upon completion of this chapter, the student should be able to:

- ▶ Identify and describe the components of assessment.
- ▶ Differentiate between objective and subjective data.
- ▶ Describe the concept of data collection and discuss the methods and sources involved in data collection.
- ▶ Discuss the importance of establishing a baseline database for comparison of future data.
- ▶ Discuss the unique characteristics of the assessment step.
- ▶ Identify modes of communication.
- ▶ Describe the purpose of therapeutic communication.
- ▶ Describe interview preparation and conducting the interview.
- ▶ Discuss the three phases of an interview.

KEY TERMS

analyze	holistic	palpation
assessment	inspection	percussion
auscultation	interpret	social communication
baseline data	interview	subjective data
closed question	objective data	therapeutic communication
closure	observation	validation
data clustering	open-ended question	verification

ASSESSMENT: STEP 1 OF THE NURSING PROCESS

Assessment is the first step in the nursing process. It involves the act of gathering data about the health status of a client (individual, resident, group of individuals). The information is collected using a systematic approach and then organized, interpreted, verified, and validated to ensure its accuracy. Finally, data are documented. The care plan is developed from assessment activities, such as the client interview and physical assessment.

> ### Nursing Tip
>
> *Data are collected from a variety of sources; however, the client should be the primary source when possible.*

Initial data collected become the foundation of the client database and are termed baseline data. Thorough and accurate data collection is an important element in planning effective client care. The professional nurse uses deliberate thought processes, judgment, and problem-solving skills as data are compiled.

Data accumulated after the initial assessment are frequently compared with baseline data to determine the client's progress or improvement or to discover trends reflecting deterioration of the client's health status.

> ### Nursing Tip
>
> *The completeness and correctness of data obtained during the interview and physical assessment are directly related to the accuracy of all steps that follow, i.e., analysis, diagnosis, and planning.*

Example: Mr. Washington, a 62-year-old African American man, is recovering from hip surgery performed 2 days ago. According to the previous staff nurse's brief report, Mr. Washington has remained stable throughout the shift. Shortly after report, Mr. Washington becomes anxious and experiences a sudden onset of dyspnea for no apparent reason. Assessment reveals tachycardia, tachypnea, and crackles in bilateral lung bases. Immediately, the nurse reviews baseline and recent vital signs along with assessment data documented during the past 24-hour nursing record. This change in Mr. Washington's condition is reported without delay to his physician. Further assessment, evaluation, and medical treatment will focus on stabilizing Mr. Washington, transferring him to the intensive care unit, and confirming the complication of pulmonary embolism.

Characteristics of Assessment

Assessment is the initial step; however, it is systematic, ongoing, and continuous. Assessment is the process of collecting data (information) to identify actual or potential health problems and strengths of the client. The data provide a sense of the client's overall health status. Data collection may include physical, psychological, social, cultural, spiritual, and cognitive areas, as well as developmental level, economic status, functional abilities, and lifestyle, depending on the tool used during data collection.

Data are gathered during an interview, physical examination, and review of diagnostic studies. Information is analyzed and validated, and facts are clustered into groups of information to identify patterns of health or illness. Assessment data are accessible to other health care team members through communication and documentation.

DATA COLLECTION

Data collection begins when the client enters the health care system. The nurse may begin collection prior to initial contact with the client through review of medical records and history. Data collection continues as long as there is a need for health care.

Types of Data

Data may be separated into two categories, subjective and objective. Subjective data, also known as *symptoms*, are statements, feelings, perceptions, or concerns communicated by a client. For example, "I'm tired" or "I'm having pain" or "I feel so afraid." Objective data, also referred to as **signs**, can be observed, measured, or felt by someone other than the person experiencing them. Table 2:1 compares subjective and objective data.

The author recommends that, as novice nurses, students separate collected data into subjective and objective data. Each category will complement and clarify the other.

> ### Nursing Tip
>
> *Subjective data reflect the client's feelings, perceptions, and concerns, stated by the client. Objective data are measurable or observable and may be acquired through physical assessment and diagnostic testing.*

TABLE 2:1 Subjective and Objective Data

Subjective	Objective
Statements, feelings, perceptions, such as: • "I'm sad." • "I feel sick to my stomach." • "I wish I were home." • "I have a burning pain in my side." • "I feel like nobody likes me." • "My heart feels like it's racing."	Data that are observable and measurable, such as: • Blood pressure of 110/70 mm Hg • Rash on right arm • Ambulates with a cane • Ate 100% of breakfast • 425 mL clear urine

Example:
- Subjective data (what the subject states): "I feel like my heart is racing."
- Objective data: Pulse 150 beats/min, regular, strong

Objective data usually support the subjective data. What the nurse observes and measures confirm what the client is feeling and experiencing. However, there may be times when objective data will conflict or seem different from what the client is stating.

Example:
- Subjective data: Client states, "I have no pain."
- Objective data: Color pale, respiratory rate increased from 18 to 26 breaths/min, clutches abdominal area

When data appear to conflict, the nurse should investigate the situation and gather all pertinent data to understand the problem.

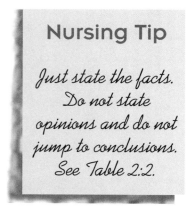

Nursing Tip

Just state the facts. Do not state opinions and do not jump to conclusions. See Table 2:2.

Sources of Data

Gathering data should involve every possible source. However, the client should be the primary source of information when possible. Family or significant others may provide useful or additional information about the client. Data may be obtained from nursing records, medical records, and verbal or written consultations. Other members of the health care team working with the client may provide valuable information. Additional sources include diagnostic results (past and present) and relevant literature, for example, accepted standards (which indicate normal functioning, such as the accepted range of a normal pulse rate).

Data Collection Tools

The assessment database should include all aspects of the client's health status. Assessment tools are designed to help nurses remember what data to collect and to organize the information obtained. Health care facilities develop preprinted documents or computerized programs, which serve as a guide for collecting and recording necessary information. Most health care facilities use assessment tools based on nursing models considered **holistic**. This term means that all aspects of the client's physical, emotional, social, spiritual, and economic well-being are considered (Figure 2:1). Otherwise, important information relating to how the client lives his or her daily life may be omitted or missed.

Some tools are organized based on problems commonly encountered on a particular nursing unit. For example, pediatric and geriatric data collection tools have additional questions pertaining to these age groups. Any format is acceptable, as long as it is thorough and comprehensive and considers the client's developmental age. Table 2:3 describes information found on various data collection tools in the client's medical record.

TABLE 2:2 Subjective and Objective Data versus Opinions and Conclusions

Subjective Data	Opinion or Conclusion
• "Don't let anyone else in my room."	• Client is angry or hostile.
• "I don't want to have that test."	• Client is anxious.
• "Get this tube out of my nose. It's killing me."	• Client is experiencing pain.
• "How do I get back to my room?"	• Client is disoriented.
• "Why hasn't the doctor seen me today?"	• Client is worried.
Objective Data	**Opinion or Conclusion**
• Dressed and shaved this morning	• Client is able to attend to ADLs (activities of daily living).
• Unsteady on feet when ambulating	• Client is intoxicated.
• Hands tremble	• Client is afraid or anxious.
• Heart rate 106 beats/min	• Client is afraid or exercising.
• Lying in dark room during the day	• Client is depressed or sad.
• Voided 300 mL amber urine	• Urine output is adequate.
• Able to change dressing to wound	• Client understands sterile technique.
• Requests pain medication every 2 hours	• Client is addicted.

Methods of Data Collection

The nurse collects data through the following methods: observation, interview, and physical assessment.

Observation

The nurse uses **observation** (the skill of watching thoughtfully and deliberately) to detect the client's overall appearance and behavior. Observations should include physical and emotional responses, moods of the client, and interaction with family or the nurse, as well as social or cultural characteristics, some of which may help or hinder data collection (Figure 2:2). These observations and others are made during initial and subsequent interactions with the client. Table 2:4 provides a checklist to aid in observation techniques.

The ability to communicate is central to the practice of nursing. It is a fundamental element in establishing a restorative nurse–client relationship. Communication includes the ability to appropriately understand, transmit, and receive thoughts,

Nursing Tip

Assessment includes collection of data, verification of accuracy, organization, interpretation, and documentation.

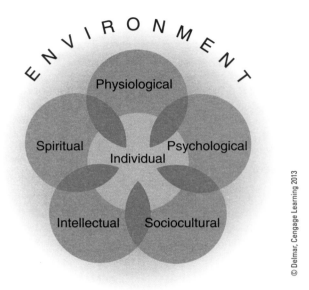

FIGURE 2:1 Holistic perspective of the individual.

TABLE 2:3 Medical Record Documents

Document	Information
Face Sheet	Biographical data: name, date of birth, address, phone number, Social Security number, marital status, employment, race, gender, religion, closest relative, insurance coverage, allergies, attending physician, admitting medical diagnosis, assigned diagnosis-related group, statement of whether the client has an advance directive
Consent Form	Admit: gives the institution and physician the right to treat Surgery: explains the reason for the operation in lay terms, the risks for complications, and the client's level of understanding Blood transfusion: permission to administer blood or blood products
Medical History and Physical Examination	Results of the client's initial history and physical assessment as performed by the health care provider
Prescriber Order Sheet	Medical orders to admit and the treatment plan
Progress Notes	Evaluation of the client's response to treatment; may contain the progress recording of interdisciplinary practitioners (e.g., dietary or social services)
Consultation Sheet	Initiated by the physician to request the evaluation or services of other practitioners

Diagnostic Sheet	Contains the results from laboratory and diagnostic tests (e.g., radiograph, hematology)
Nursing Assessment	Recording of data obtained from the interview and physical assessment conducted by the nurse
Nursing Plan of Care	Contains the treatment plan (e.g., nursing diagnosis or a problem list, initiation of standards of care or protocols)
Graphic Sheet	Data recording regarding vital signs and weight
Flow Sheet	Contains all routine interventions that can be noted with a check mark or other simple codes; allows for a quick comparison of measurement
Nurse's Progress Notes	Additional data that do not duplicate information on the flow sheet (e.g., client's achievement of expected outcome or revision of the plan of care)
Medication Administration Record	Contains all medication information for routine and prn (as needed) drugs: date, time, dose, route, site (for injections)
Patient Education Record	Recording of the nurses' teaching to the client, family, or other caregiver and the learner's response
Health Care Team Record	Treatment and progress record for nonmedical and nonnursing practitioners, when the physician's progress notes are not used by other practitioners (e.g., respiratory, physical therapy, dietary)
Clinical Pathway	A multidisciplinary form for each day of anticipated hospitalization that identifies the interventions and achievement of client outcomes; the practitioner's initial implementation and variances from the norm are explained in the progress notes
Discharge Plan and Summary	A multidisciplinary form used before discharge from a health care facility containing a brief summary of care rendered and discharge instructions (e.g., food–drug interactions, referrals, or follow-up appointments)
Advance Directive or Living Will	Federal law requires that health care providers discuss with clients the use of advance directives, commonly known as the living will or durable power of attorney; most states recognize the living will as a legal document; if the client has advance directives, they are reviewed at the time of admission and placed in the medical record

Source: Delaune, Sue C., & Ladner, Patricia K. (2011). *Fundamentals of Nursing: Standards and Practice* (4th ed.) New York: Cengage Learning.

Use your senses of observation

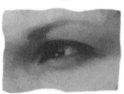 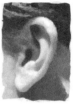 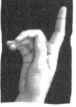

LOOK   **LISTEN**   **FEEL**   **SMELL**

Note the client's overall general appearance - Thin?
Obese? Well-groomed? Does the client look his or her
stated age?

Note body language or posture. How is the client sitting?
Is the client withdrawing? Is he or she making eye contact?
Observe the client's facial expressions.

Be aware of your method of interaction. Are you too close?
Too far away? Remember cultural differences.

© Delmar, Cengage Learning 2013

FIGURE 2:2

feelings, and facts. In addition, nurses must be aware of cultural differences and variances related to communication. When cultural variances exist, inaccurate interpretation of communication may occur. Table 2:5 describes ways of overcoming possible cultural communication barriers.

Interview

An interview is a communication exchange between the client and nurse. This exchange has a specific purpose, which is to collect information about the client. Discoveries relating to the client's

TABLE 2:4 Aids to Observation

- Use your senses _____
- Note the client's general appearance _____
  _____
- Note body language _____
  _____
- Be aware of own interaction patterns _____
  Remember cultural differences relating to behavior.

TABLE 2:5 Overcoming Cultural Communication Barriers

- When the client and nurse speak different languages, obtain an interpreter to facilitate communication.
- Even though a client of a different culture and a nurse may speak the same language, verify the client's understanding of the exchange. Words may have different meanings to different people.
- Nonverbal communication, such as facial expression, posture, gestures, lack of eye contact, and use of silence, are communication variances often misinterpreted.
- Consider social and family relationships, religion, language, food, and cultural view of health or illness when working with clients from differing cultures.
- Maintain a nonjudgmental attitude.
- Recognize biases.

present and past health status allow the nurse to make determinations and decisions about health needs. Nurses use knowledge of communication to discerningly obtain facts and information. This information is gathered through conversation and observations during the structured interview. Developing interviewing skills takes time and practice.

There are different types of communication: therapeutic and social. For the purpose of data collection, the nurse uses therapeutic communication. This interaction results in conversations with a client, which are neither idle nor meaningless, but purposeful, goal-directed, client-focused, and planned. Social communication is casual conversation, spontaneous, and with no planned agenda.

Nursing Tip

People differ in many ways:
- Age
- Gender
- Educational level
- Language
- Occupation
- Residence (rural, urban, suburban)
- Socioeconomic status
- Religion
- Functional abilities
- Cognitive abilities
- Racial composition
- Nationality
- Family structure and ties

Interview Preparation

Preparation and planning are key to effective interviewing. Suggestions for preparation include reviewing medical records, reviewing current admission documentation of past or present client care, and researching present and past medical diagnoses. In addition, forethought should be given to strategies for overcoming potential communication barriers that might impede successful data collection during the interview process. Table 2:6 identifies common barriers to therapeutic interaction.

TABLE 2:6 Barriers to Therapeutic Interaction

Barrier	Example
• Language differences	• Difficulty navigating through health care system.
	• Prevents evaluation of client's response to nursing interventions.
• Sociocultural differences	• Use of language may differ from nurse. Interpretation of words may be different.
• Gender	• Communication can vary between men and women.
• Health status	• The disoriented or confused client may be unable to reliably communicate.
	• Alterations in sensory or perceptual function, such as impairment or loss of vision, hearing, or sense of touch, affect the ability to send or receive communication messages.
	• Moderate to severe pain or discomfort and other health-related difficulties, such as dyspnea, may impair communication.
• Developmental level	• May require a different approach, different language, or different terminology for a client (e.g., a child) to understand.
• Knowledge differences	• Client and family may have varying levels of education. Listen to conversations and vocabulary chosen. Consider the client's mental capabilities.
• Emotional distance	• Therapeutic communication involves establishing a caring, empathetic relationship with the client. Emotional distance refers to a barrier existing between the client and nurse that prevents effective therapeutic communication. Examples include a client in respiratory isolation or a comatose or confused client.
• Emotions	• Fear, anxiety, and depression are examples of emotions that prevent therapeutic communication.
• Daydreaming	• Allowing one's mind to wander instead of being an active listener may lead to missing the point of the message. Nurses must be attentive, alert, and focused on the conversation.

Conducting the Interview

The interview most often occurs at the beginning of the nurse–client relationship. The nurse may institute various techniques in an effort to build rapport with the client (Figure 2:3). Rapport promotes positive interactions between the health care team and client.

Techniques that advocate productive, therapeutic communication include active listening, conveying acceptance, being attentive, sitting at eye level with the client (if possible), and establishing eye-to-eye contact.

Controlling the environment, making it more conducive for the interview, is an important part of preparation. This includes providing privacy, allowing adequate time for answering questions, maintaining a comfortable room temperature, reducing environmental noise levels, and eliminating or decreasing distractions, if possible.

Data collection is facilitated by various communication techniques. During the interview, nurses ask questions to elicit a particular response. How questions are asked will determine client responses (Figure 2:4). Open-ended questions are stated in a manner that encourages the client to elaborate about a particular concern or problem. For example, "What types of food do you usually eat during a 24-hour period?" or "What led to your coming here today?" Each of these questions encourages the client to respond with information. Closed questions can be answered with brief yes-or-no answers. This type of questioning may be appropriate in certain situations, for example, in an emergency: "Did she respond to you when you entered her room?" or "How many pounds has she lost over the last month?" Additional techniques that promote communication during an interview or therapeutic nurse–client communication can be found in Table 2:7 and Figure 2:5.

Tips to help you establish rapport with the client

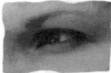

MAINTAIN EYE CONTACT

1. Interview in a private setting - environment should be quiet, private. Turn down the TV. Close the room door.

2. When addressing the client, use appropriate title. Introduce yourself.

3. State the purpose of the exchange/interview. Explain why you will be asking questions.

4. Maintain eye contact - do not stare but be attentive.

5. Do not rush through the data collection tool. Use a caring, interested manner, clarifying and investigating, when appropriate.

© Delmar, Cengage Learning, 2013

FIGURE 2:3

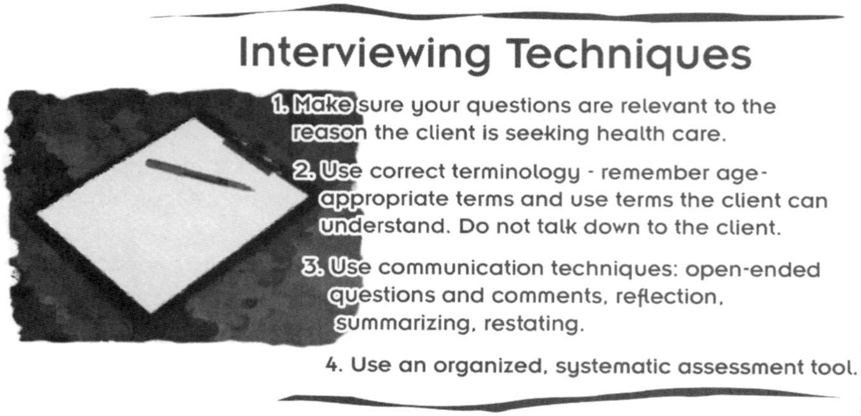

Interviewing Techniques

1. Make sure your questions are relevant to the reason the client is seeking health care.

2. Use correct terminology - remember age-appropriate terms and use terms the client can understand. Do not talk down to the client.

3. Use communication techniques: open-ended questions and comments, reflection, summarizing, restating.

4. Use an organized, systematic assessment tool.

© Delmar, Cengage Learning, 2013

FIGURE 2:4

TABLE 2:7 Therapeutic Communication Techniques

Paraphrasing	Restate what was said by the sender in the receiver's own words to make sure the statement was understood accurately.
Clarifying	Asking the sender to restate an unclear message or to give an example will allow confirmation of whether or not the message was interpreted correctly.
Focusing	When the sender introduces more than one unrelated topic in the same conversation or when the discussion becomes unclear, the receiver redirects the conversation back to a specific topic.
Summarizing	Reviewing a conversation and focusing on key issues provide a synopsis of the main ideas from the discussion.
Responses and Actions to Avoid	<ul><li>Inattentive listening, such as breaking eye contact, glancing around the room, or fidgeting, conveys the message that what the sender has to say is not important.</li><li>Using unfamiliar medical terminology may be confusing to the patient and family.</li><li>Asking unrelated personal questions simply to satisfy your curiosity is inappropriate.</li><li>Providing false reassurance may discourage expression of feelings.</li><li>Inappropriate socializing borders on unprofessional behavior and blocks therapeutic communication.</li><li>Passive responses sidestep subject matter or conflict.</li><li>Aggressive responses trigger conflict.</li></ul>

Promoting a Successful Interview

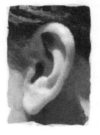

LISTEN!

1. Listen actively! Convey acceptance - make eye contact, nod your head to show interest. Be attentive - concentrate on the client's words.

2. Allow client/family member to finish his or her thoughts and sentences - don't interrupt.

3. Be patient - allow time for client to answer or respond.

4. When appropriate, summarize and restate.

© Delmar, Cengage Learning, 2013

FIGURE 2:5

Bringing Closure to the Interview

The nurse should indicate in some manner that the interview session is coming to an end. For example, the nurse could state that most of the information has been collected and only a few more facts are necessary. During closure, the nurse allows the client to present additional relevant information and then summarizes overall information that has been covered or accomplished. The nurse determines if additional sessions will be necessary for further exploration and, if so, plans are made with the client.

Physical Examination

The purpose of a physical examination is to collect data regarding the client's present health status and to establish a baseline physical assessment. Direct observations can be made that may indicate deviations from normal. Validation and clarification of any subjective complaint may be obtained.

REFLECTION   ASSESSING

A nursing student is assigned to provide care to a 74-year-old man whose admitting diagnosis is an abscess formed in the epidural region after thoracic surgery (2 months ago). After receiving long-term antibiotics with little improvement, magnetic resonance imaging was ordered, and an abscess was discovered. He was admitted yesterday for further evaluation and treatment. The patient's past medical history includes diabetes, hypertension, and hyperlipidemia.

Where does one begin with such a client? First things first . . . that is, *assessment* begins the nursing process. Recall that activities involved in the assessment step include data collection, that is, communication with the primary nurse or others involved in the client's care, review of previous and current patient data, observation at the bedside, interviewing or talking with the client, and performing a physical assessment.

Baseline and current data may be found in the client's chart or electronic medical record. Look over demographic data, allergies, code status, and past and current level of functioning. Review admission orders, such as prescribed diet, activity level, wound care, and additional facts, that aid in the understanding of the client's current health care needs. Next, use purposeful communication techniques to interview the client. As the dialogue ensues with the review of systems, the student will apply the skill of observation.

- Look for signs of distress (e.g., pallor, labored breathing, emotional distress, guarding behavior indicating pain).
- Scan the room for safety hazards (side rails, height of bed, spills or clutter on floor).
- Look at the equipment in the client's room (e.g., urinary catheter and characteristics of the urine in the collection bag, intravenous pumps, rate and fluids infusing, oxygen, suction devices, monitors).
- Observe how persons in the room interact with the client.
- Observe the client closely (e.g., position of body, skin characteristics, intravenous site, breathing effort, condition of the bed linens).
- Observe the wound for drainage, odor, and condition of wound dressing.
- Perform a systematic nursing physical assessment of all body systems using inspection, auscultation, percussion, and palpation techniques. Record data in a retrievable format. Use factual, concrete, specific terms.
- Avoid vague statements, such as "tolerated well," "normal," or "good"

Nursing Tip

- Always promote communication while assessing.
- Ask questions and then allow time for response.
- Do not rely on memory. Write it down.
- Choose a method for organizing your assessment, e.g., head to toe, body systems.

During a physical examination, the nurse uses various techniques to collect data. Initial physical data collected, known as baseline data, are documented and used for comparison and evaluation of the client's status at a given point in time.

Physical Examination Techniques

Physical assessment techniques include *inspection, auscultation, palpation,* and *percussion*. A brief description of each technique follows.

Inspection is a systematic process of observation that includes vision. Through sight, the nurse observes skin color and condition and notes drainage, the effort to breathe, and respiratory pattern. Inspection includes noting one's body posture, gait, ability to use extremities, and facial expressions or observing the client's ability to carry out activities of daily living (ADLs).

- Use a penlight or natural or artificial lighting to enhance inspection.
- Maintain privacy during inspection and throughout all phases of the physical examination.
- Explain the inspection technique to the client prior to beginning to reduce anxiety.

Auscultation is the technique of listening for sounds within the body, usually with a stethoscope. Areas most often auscultated include the lungs, heart, abdomen, and blood vessels.

Palpation is an assessment technique involving use of touch or pressing on the external surface of the body with the fingers. Palpation is used to assess texture, temperature, moisture of the skin, organ location and size, vibrations and pulsations, swelling, masses, and tenderness. Examples of uses of palpation include:

- Touch: may be used to detect a mass, conditions of the skin, e.g., moisture, dryness, and skin temperature
- Pressure: may be used to feel the quality and rate of an arterial pulsation, determine capillary refill, assess skin turgor, or evaluate for edema
- Deep palpation: may be used for assessment of deep, internal organ anomalies or to determine if the client is experiencing an abnormal response to pain

Percussion is the technique involving direct or indirect tapping of a specific body surface to glean information about internal organs beneath the body surface. The health care provider may use fingertips, fist, or percussion hammer to elicit various tones indicating the presence or absence of fluid or air, masses, consolidation, tenderness, and normal or abnormal reflexes.

Nursing Tip

Assessment begins with the first encounter of the client. Data are collected during the initial interview and physical examination. Each interaction with the client is an opportunity for assessment and data collection.

DATA VERIFICATION AND VALIDATION

After all data are gathered, information is **verified** (confirmed or proved) and **validated** (determined to be fact) to ensure accuracy. Data are reviewed for omissions, inconsistencies, and possible inaccuracies. For example, a confused client is admitted to the medical surgical unit, stating that he has no family. However, you were told that the person who brought him in was his wife. In another example, a client may state that he ambulates without difficulty and without the use of assistive devices. The client's wife states he uses a cane. The nurse observes the client ambulating with an unsteady gait. In each case, the nurse would need to consider possible reasons for the discrepancy and collect more information before forming conclusions and planning care.

Nursing Tip

Identify problems by asking the following questions:

1. Has the client experienced any change in his or her usual functional pattern?

2. Has the client demonstrated any indication of abnormal functioning of a body system?

3. Has the client demonstrated deviation from normal range compared with standards?

INTERPRETATION AND ORGANIZATION OF DATA

Data that have been collected, verified, and validated for accuracy are now ready to be **analyzed** (processing information to reach a conclusion) and **interpreted** (determining the meaning and significance). For this process, the nurse assigns meaning to collected data and groups data into clusters. Data are compared against standards such as normal health patterns, normal vital signs, lab values, basic food groups, or normal growth and development. Interpreting and analyzing data help identify missing information or inconsistencies. After these have been identified, it is necessary to gather more data.

Data clustering is the process of organizing subjective and objective data into groups of related cues. This process is used to determine the relatedness of facts, to find patterns, and to determine if further data are needed. Ultimately, data clustering assists in identifying areas of health care deviations requiring treatment or support.

Example:

1. "Reports sudden onset of abdominal pain rated 6 on a scale of 0 to 10, observed facial mask of pain, guarding abdominal area" are clustered data indicating acute pain as a nursing diagnosis.
2. "Reports difficulty carrying out ADLs, observed difficulty dressing self and brushing hair" are clustered data indicating problems with self-care abilities.
3. "Uses a walker, has difficulty ambulating, stumbles and looses balance when attempting to ambulate to bathroom" are clustered data indicating problems with mobility.

DOCUMENTING ASSESSMENT DATA

Documentation of data collected during the assessment is essential. Documentation is the process of preparing a record that reflects the assessment data and describes the client's present health status. When documenting this information, the nurse communicates with others involved in the client's care. This is necessary to provide quality care.

Various formats are utilized for documentation, depending on the agency. Data may be documented using narrative or electronic notations, checklists, a combination of the two, or specialty formats. Chapter 5 discusses and describes different types of documentation.

KEY CONCEPTS

- Assessment is the first step in the nursing process. Information is gathered through an interview, physical examination, and review of diagnostic tests. These data reveal a sense of the overall health status of the client.
- Assessment is ongoing throughout the nursing process sequence.
- During assessment, data are collected, organized, interpreted, verified, validated, and then documented.
- The care plan is developed from and based on data collected during initial and ongoing assessment.
- Two types of data are collected: subjective and objective. Generally, each category will complement and clarify the other.
- The client should be the primary source of information. When this is not possible, family or significant others may provide useful or additional information about the client.
- Data sources include the client, nursing records, medical records, verbal and written consultations, diagnostic results, and relevant literature.

- Methods of data collection include observation, interview, and physical examination.
- Collected data should be verified and validated to ensure accuracy. Data should be reviewed for omissions and incongruities. If these are discovered, possible reasons for the discrepancy or inaccuracy should be identified and corrected.
- Clustering helps to organize data and determine the *relatedness* of subjective and objective information. Clustering also aids in finding patterns. This technique provides confirmation that an identified problem exists and should be included in the care plan.

STUDENT PRACTICE: DEVELOPING COMMUNICATION AND DATA COLLECTION

Instructions

Provide responses to the following:

1. Define *baseline database* and explain its importance. _____

   _____

   _____

2. Define *subjective* and *objective data*. Provide an example of each. _____

   _____

   _____

3. List characteristics of therapeutic communication. _____

   _____

   _____

4. Describe communication techniques that promote therapeutic communication. _____

   _____

   _____

5. Explain the role of the interview, observation, and physical assessment in data collection. _____

   _____

   _____

   _____

6. List key elements of a successful interview. _____

   _____

   _____

STUDENT PRACTICE: DEVELOPING OPEN-ENDED QUESTIONS

Instructions

Transform the following closed questions to open-ended questions or comments to promote therapeutic communication.

1. "Are you feeling better?"

   _____

   _____

2. "Did you like the dinner?"

   _____

   _____

3. "Are you in pain?"

   _____

   _____

4. "Do you understand what the doctor told you about the surgery?"

   _____

   _____

5. "Do you understand the doctor's instructions?"

   _____

   _____

STUDENT PRACTICE: DEVELOPING THERAPEUTIC COMMUNICATION TECHNIQUES

Instructions

Rewrite the following quotes using specified therapeutic communication techniques:

1. The client comments, "Nothing ever goes right for me." Use reflection and write your response.

   _____

   _____

   _____

2. The client is extremely quiet and avoids eye contact. Use observation and write your response.

_____

_____

_____

3. The client states, "They told me I had to have surgery. I'm so afraid. I couldn't sleep last night. I'm waiting for my husband to call me from home. He had to pick up the kids. Right now, I have a headache." Use focusing and write your response. _____

_____

_____

4. The client states, "I felt full even before I started eating." Use clarifying and write your response.

_____

_____

_____

STUDENT PRACTICE: IDENTIFYING OBJECTIVE AND SUBJECTIVE DATA

Instructions

Underline *abnormal* data discovered in the situations below. List subjective and objective data.

Scenario: Cherisha Martin, a 56-year-old African American woman, was seen at the clinic with multiple urinary system complaints. She reports that her urine is cloudy, is amber colored, and has a pungent odor. She has an urge to urinate more frequently; however, she voids small amounts. Two days ago, she saw blood in her urine. Her vital signs are blood pressure, 142/92 mm Hg; pulse rate, 78 beats/min and regular; respirations, 20 breaths/min; and temperature, 100.4°F.

1. List abnormal subjective data from the case scenario above.

_____

_____

_____

2. List abnormal objective data from the case scenario above.

_____

_____

_____

Scenario: Richardo Gutierrez, a 34-year-old Hispanic man, was involved in a roll-over motor vehicle accident 1 day ago. In the accident, he sustained a crushing injury to his right hand. He has multiple superficial cuts from broken glass on his arms and face. This morning he describes his hand pain as throbbing and deep. He rates his pain as a 6 on a 0 to 10 scale. The dressing on his hand is intact with a small amount of dry, reddish-brown drainage observed in the palmar region. His fingertips are edematous and warm with a brisk capillary refill. His radial pulse is palpable and within normal limits.

1. List abnormal subjective data from the case scenario above.

   _____

   _____

   _____

2. List abnormal objective data from the case scenario above.

   _____

   _____

   _____

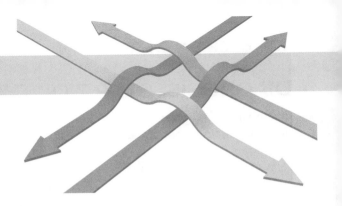

CHAPTER 3

DIAGNOSIS

OBJECTIVES

Upon completion of this chapter, the student should be able to:

▶ Identify characteristics of nursing diagnoses.

▶ Identify and discuss differences between medical and nursing diagnoses.

▶ Describe the different types of nursing diagnoses.

▶ List components of actual and risk nursing diagnoses.

▶ Describe the process of developing a nursing diagnosis.

KEY TERMS

actual nursing diagnosis
defining characteristics
diagnosis
etiology

medical diagnosis
nursing diagnosis
problem
problem statement

risk nursing diagnosis
wellness diagnosis

DIAGNOSIS: STEP 2 OF THE NURSING PROCESS

Diagnosis is the second phase of the nursing process. It involves the classification of disease, condition, or human response based upon scientific evaluation of signs, symptoms, history, and diagnostic studies. *Diagnosis* is also referred to as *analysis, problem identification,* or *nursing diagnosis.* These corresponding terms are used interchangeably.

During the assessment phase, nurses use critical-thinking skills and judgment to analyze, organize, and interpret assessment data. Problems, potential problems, and strengths of the client are identified. In the diagnosis phase, problems, potential problems, and strengths are labeled with an appropriate **nursing diagnosis**. After they are labeled, the nursing diagnosis communicates specific health care needs about the client to other members of the health care team involved in care.

Nursing Tip

All activities preceding this phase are directed toward formulating the nursing diagnosis, i.e., problem identification. All care planning activities following this phase are based on the nursing diagnosis, the identified problem(s).

Differentiating between Medical and Nursing Diagnoses

A medical diagnosis is made by the physician or advance health care practitioner and refers to a disease, condition, or pathological state only a practitioner can treat. Examples of medical diagnoses are diabetes mellitus, congestive heart failure, hepatitis, cancer, and pneumonia. The medical diagnosis usually does not change. Nurses are required to follow the physician's order(s) and carry out prescribed treatments and therapies.

The term *nursing diagnosis* is used in three different contexts. First, it refers to the distinct second step in the nursing process, diagnosis. Next, nursing diagnosis applies to the label. Nurses assign meaning to collected assessment data. Actual problems and problems the client is at risk for developing are identified and appropriately labeled with a North American Nursing Diagnosis

Association (NANDA)-approved nursing diagnosis. For example, a client is admitted into the hospital and medically treated for a heart attack (acute myocardial infarction). The physician prescribes treatment, such as diagnostic tests, therapies, and various medications. The nurse carries out the physician orders and monitors the client. During the assessment, the nurse may identify that the client is experiencing anxiety over the medical diagnosis, fear and anxiety over an uncertain future, and difficulty sleeping. It is those problems that are labeled with nursing diagnoses: respectively, *Anxiety, Fear,* and *Sleep Pattern Disturbed.* Nurses will intervene individually or collectively with the physician to resolve each response. Nurses understand the holistic needs of the client and use scientific knowledge, insight, and critical thought as physician-prescribed treatment and nursing interventions are carried out. Finally, a nursing diagnosis refers to one of many diagnoses in the classification system established and approved by NANDA.

Characteristics of Nursing Diagnoses

Actual nursing diagnoses describe the client's response to a physical, sociocultural, psychological, or spiritual illness, disease, or condition. Actual signs and symptoms are present. For example, the physician diagnoses a client with a medical illness, pneumonia, and writes orders for hospital admission and treatment. During the initial interview and physical health assessment, subjective and objective data are collected indicating that the client is restless, hypoxic (reduced oxygen in inspired air), and too weak to cough productively. The nurse correctly identifies and labels one nursing diagnosis as *Impaired Gas Exchange.* Interventions will be planned and instituted by the nurse to improve the client's gas exchange at the cellular level, aiding in problem improvement or resolution.

Nursing diagnoses may communicate possible developing problems resulting from a client's physical, sociocultural, psychological, or spiritual illness, disease, or condition, termed **risk nursing diagnoses**. For example, an elderly client experiencing vertigo and difficulty walking but refuses to call for assistance with ambulation. The appropriate potential problem would be identified and labeled as *Risk for Injury.*

Nursing diagnoses may change as the client's condition improves or the problem resolves or becomes worse. Refer to the example of the client diagnosed with *Impaired Gas Exchange.* Nurses carry out physician-prescribed treatment for pneumonia, for example, administer antibiotics, provide hydration, and so on, and the client's physical condition improves. One would expect gas exchange within the lungs to improve. In this case, the problem of *Impaired Gas Exchange* would probably be resolved.

Nursing diagnoses may complement physician-prescribed treatment but are separate and distinct. For example, if the hospitalized client had undergone a surgical procedure, one would expect to find physician-ordered analgesics. Medication is one important method to treat pain. (See Table 3:1, which shows an example of an analgesic order that a physician would write.) There are also many independent nonpharmacological nursing interventions that may be initiated to alleviate the client's pain, and that would complement physician-prescribed treatment. Examples include imagery, distraction, relaxation, and massage.

TABLE 3:1 Determining Appropriate Interventions Using Critical Thought

Mrs. Johnson, 66 years of age, is admitted after falling and fracturing her pelvis. Data are gathered through an interview and physical assessment. The client requests medication for pain. The pain she is experiencing is a physiological response to her injury. Using a NANDA nursing diagnosis, the response is labeled as *Acute Pain*.

Mrs. Johnson's physician has written analgesic orders, as follows:

- Demerol 50 mg, intramuscular, every 4 hours, as needed for severe pain
- Vicodin one or two, by mouth, every 4 hours, as needed for moderate pain
- Tylenol ES two, by mouth, every 4 hours, as needed for mild pain

What decision-making questions should the nurse ask Mrs. Johnson regarding her pain?

Nursing Tip

A client's medical diagnosis remains the same for as long as the disease process is present, but nursing diagnoses often change as the client's responses change.

Actual nursing diagnoses are developed when an *existing response* to an illness, a disease, or a condition is present at the time of the nursing assessment. The problem actually exists. The client is demonstrating subjective or objective data to support the conclusion. Actual nursing diagnoses are based on the presence of associated signs and symptoms.

Examples:

Hyperthermia, client's temperature is 104.6°F
Impaired Gas Exchange, client's oxygen saturation in arterial blood is 92%
Pain, client states pain level is 8 on a scale of 0 to 10
Anxiety, client states he is experiencing anxiety
Self-Care Deficit, client is unable to perform ADLs

Risk diagnoses are determined when a possible problem may develop but has not yet occurred. NANDA defines risk diagnosis as "a clinical judgment made when a client is more vulnerable to develop the problem than others in the same or similar situations."

Example:

Any person admitted into the hospital is at risk for acquiring a nosocomial infection. However, a client medically diagnosed with cancer, who is receiving chemotherapy and whose immune system is depressed, will hold a higher risk than others will for developing a hospital-acquired infection. The nurse would appropriately label this potential problem as *Risk for Infection*. After the problem has been identified, the health care team can take deliberate action and initiate interventions to prevent the problem from occurring.

Example:

An active 80-year-old woman was admitted into the hospital 2 days ago after falling in her home and sustaining a hip fracture. On day 1 after surgical repair, the client is experiencing a great deal of pain and refuses to move. Immobility, advanced age, and the client's refusal to shift her weight place the client at a greater risk for developing pressure ulcers. The nurse appropriately labels this potential problem as *Risk for Impaired Skin Integrity* and plans interventions to prevent skin breakdown from occurring.

Components of Actual Nursing Diagnoses

For *actual* nursing diagnoses, the **problem statement** consists of three components: problem, etiology, and defining characteristics. Each element has a specific purpose.

The **problem** is the identified label of a client's health condition or response to the medical illness or therapy for which nursing may intervene. The problem is also known as the nursing diagnosis.

The **etiology**, written as "related to" (*R/T*) includes conditions most likely to be involved in the development of a problem. This factor becomes the focus for nursing interventions. The etiology or cause component of the nursing diagnosis identifies one or more probable causes of the abnormal response. The etiology gives direction to the problem statement. In view of this fact, the nurse is able to individualize care. NANDA uses the term *related factor* to describe the etiology or likely cause of the actual nursing diagnosis.

> ## Nursing Tip
>
> - *The same set of nursing diagnoses cannot be expected to occur with a particular disease or condition.*
> - *A single nursing diagnosis may occur as a response to any number of diseases.*

REFLECTION DIAGNOSING

Mrs. Throng, an 83-year-old Vietnamese woman, was admitted with a medical diagnosis of pneumonia. During the *assessment* phase, data were collected and documented. The next step of the nursing process is *diagnosing*. During this step, the nurse analyzes and interprets previously collected data. Mrs. Throng was found to have bilateral lung congestion, moderate fever, chills, an aching chest, generalized weakness, dyspnea, and a productive cough. She has had no appetite for almost 1 week. The chest radiograph showed areas of consolidation. Her oxygen saturation is low (92%) but within an acceptable range. All other assessment findings were unremarkable.

Now that data collection is complete, data will be organized and analyzed. Group together data that seem related, such as bilateral lung congestion, productive cough, and chest x-ray consolidation. Additional findings that seem to support this cluster of cues include dyspnea and low oxygen saturation. Determine the meaning of data clusters. How can the cluster of cues be labeled in a way that all other nurses understand?

In Mrs. Throng's case, at least one or more actual problems exist indicating a need for nursing assistance. Certainly, abnormal responses place an emphasis on the respiratory system. Appropriate nursing diagnoses to be included in the plan of care are:

- Impaired Gas Exchange: related to decreased functional lung tissue, ventilation–perfusion imbalance, as evidenced by dyspnea, hypoxemia, and O_2 saturation of 92%
- Ineffective Airway Clearance: related to inflammation and the presence of secretions, as evidenced by chest x-ray consolidation, productive cough, and abnormal lung sounds

Remember . . . as a nursing student, when a possible nursing diagnosis is identified and thought to be appropriate to add to the plan of care, always begin by reading the definition of the nursing diagnosis first.

Nursing Tip

Remember, for actual nursing diagnoses, there are subjective or objective data, evidence that the problem actually exists.

Defining characteristics, written "as evidenced by" (AEB), are the clinical signs and symptoms that confirm the problem is occurring. This component reflects *how* the diagnosis or problematic response is manifested.

Student Practice Examples

The following scenarios describe patient situations in which clinical signs and symptoms resulting from their illness, condition, or injury are exhibited. The actual nursing diagnosis is provided.

A. Using a nursing diagnosis handbook, locate the nursing diagnosis and read the definition.
B. List all appropriate "related to" and "as evidenced by" components.

Scenario one: The nurse is caring for a client who was involved in a motor vehicle accident and sustained superficial skin trauma. The client's epidermal layer of skin on the right knee, forearm, and hand is excoriated, reddened, and bleeding as the result of sliding across a cement pavement. (*Impaired Skin Integrity*)

_____

_____

_____

_____

_____

Scenario two: Carson, a 2-year-old boy, has had a productive cough for 3 days. His respiratory rate is increased for his age, and he is irritable. Carson is diagnosed with acute bronchitis and placed on antibiotics and home breathing treatments. (*Impaired Gas Exchange*)

Scenario three: The client you are caring for has been medically diagnosed with a right cerebral vascular accident (stroke). He experiences partial paralysis on the left side of his body. He is unable to turn over while in bed without assistance and has demonstrated decreased muscle strength and control in the left extremities. (*Impaired Physical Mobility*)

Components of Risk Nursing Diagnoses

Risk nursing diagnoses are identified when the client is *at risk* for developing a problem. The problem statement consists of two components, the problem and risk factor. The term *risk factor* is used to describe the etiology of risk nursing diagnoses because there are no subjective or objective data present. The actual problem *does not exist* at the time of assessment. However, because of clinical circumstances, the client is at risk for developing this specific problem or complication. Table 3:3 compares components of actual and risk nursing diagnoses.

> ### Nursing Tip
> Differentiating among possible causes of an identified problem is essential. Each cause or etiology may require different nursing interventions (see Table 3:2).

Examples of Risk Nursing Diagnoses

- Cancer patient, *Risk for Infection*
  R/T: inadequate secondary defenses, immunosuppression
- Client with surgical incision, *Risk for Infection*
  R/T: inadequate primary defenses, invasive procedure
- Client who is semiconscious and vomiting, *Risk for Aspiration*
  R/T: reduced level of consciousness, vomiting

TABLE 3:2 Comparison of Same Nursing Diagnoses with Different Etiologies Requiring Different Interventions

Nursing Diagnosis	Client	Etiology	Nursing Interventions
Constipation, Perceived	Jim Beason	Inactivity, insufficient fiber intake	• Encourage daily activity to stimulate bowel elimination. • Teach components of high-fiber diet to improve bowel function.
	Terry Fielder	Long-term laxative use	• Identify factors that may contribute to constipation, such as medications, reduced fluid intake, and dietary habits. • Instruct client on adverse effects of long-term laxative use.
Ineffective Breast-feeding	Christi Lawrence	Inadequate sucking reflex in infant	• Assess infant's ability to latch on and suck effectively. • Monitor maternal skill with latching infant onto the nipple.
	Cheri Phillips	Inexperience, knowledge deficit	• Determine mother's desire and motivation to breastfeed. • Evaluate mother's understanding of infant's feeding cues, such as rooting.

TABLE 3:3 Comparison of Components in Actual and Risk Nursing Diagnoses

Actual Nursing Diagnosis	Risk Nursing Diagnosis
Three components: • Nursing diagnosis • Related factor(s) • Defining characteristics	Two components: • Risk nursing diagnosis • Risk factor(s)

Nursing Tip

For risk nursing diagnoses, there are no defining characteristics or AEB per se. R/T identifies characteristics that make the client more vulnerable to developing a specific problem.

- Neonate unable to maintain his body temperature; parent does not keep the child covered, *Risk for Hypothermia*
  R/T: extremes of age, inadequate clothing
- Unsteady gait, refuses to call for assistance, *Risk for Injury*
  R/T: impaired mobility, lack of knowledge regarding safety precautions

Wellness Nursing Diagnoses

NANDA defines wellness diagnosis as "a clinical judgment about an individual, family, or community in transition from a specific level of wellness to a higher level of wellness." Wellness nursing diagnoses require a one-part statement, for example, *Readiness for Enhanced Nutrition* (client has expressed a desire for improved nutritional status).

KEY CONCEPTS

- Diagnosis is the second step in the nursing process.
- Nursing diagnoses are different than medical diagnoses in that nursing diagnoses describe the *client's response* to a physical, sociocultural, psychological, or spiritual illness, disease, or condition.
- Nurses have legal and ethical responsibilities to both medical and nursing diagnoses.
- Nursing diagnoses may change as the client's health status changes.
- The two most common nursing diagnoses are *actual* and *risk* nursing diagnoses.
- An actual nursing diagnosis includes three components: the problem (nursing diagnosis label), etiology (related to), and defining characteristics (as evidenced by).
- A risk nursing diagnosis includes two components: the potential problem (risk nursing diagnosis) and risk factors (related to).
- Wellness nursing diagnoses require a one-part statement. Wellness nursing diagnoses may be included in the care plan for individuals expressing desire for a higher level of wellness.

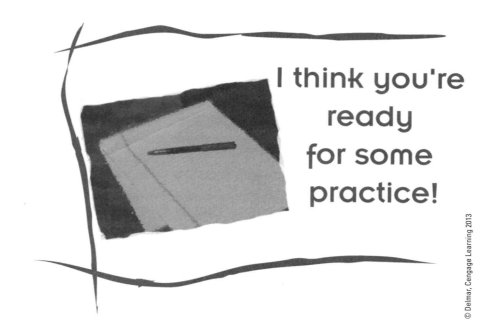

I think you're ready for some practice!

STUDENT PRACTICE: WRITING DIAGNOSIS STATEMENTS

Instructions

Read each case history and follow directions.

A. *Underline* abnormal subjective data and circle abnormal objective data.
B. Complete the *three-part* diagnostic statement that clearly describes the nursing diagnosis. In other words, what is the *R/T* and *AEB* information you will include with the nursing diagnosis?

1. Carl James was hospitalized yesterday. Today he demonstrates the following signs and symptoms: blood pressure, 138/78 mm Hg; pulse rate, 102 beats/min and regular; respiratory rate, 24 breaths/min and using accessory muscles; restless; and irritable. Oral temperature is 99.8°F. The pulse oximeter reading is 94%. Mr. James is diaphoretic and complains of a headache. His lung sounds are clear but diminished. He states he feels "light-headed" when he moves from his bed to the chair. (Nursing diagnosis, *Impaired Gas Exchange*)

_____

_____

_____

_____

2. Mrs. Silverman has recently completed chemotherapy and radiation for breast cancer. She arrived at the clinic this morning with the following signs and symptoms: no appetite, weight loss of 4 pounds since her last visit 2 weeks ago, and nausea without vomiting. She states that most of the time she feels exhausted. "The inside of my mouth hurts," she says. Assessment reveals oral ulcerations that are erythematous (reddened). Her vital signs are within normal range. (Nursing diagnosis, *Imbalanced Nutrition: Less Than Body Requirements*)

3. Kam Le returned from South America 1 week ago. He has experienced nausea, vomiting, and diarrhea for 4 days and exhibits the following additional symptoms: inelastic skin turgor, dry oral mucous membranes, weakness, and an elevated temperature. (Nursing diagnosis, *Fluid Volume Deficient*)

4. Seventy-seven-year-old Hilda Jameson is being evaluated at the clinic. Her daughter states that Mrs. Jameson has not been as active as usual and has experienced frequent episodes of confusion. Examination confirms that she is disoriented to time and place and asks that someone find her husband. Her daughter reports that he has been deceased for several years. (Nursing diagnosis, *Disturbed Thought Processes*)

STUDENT PRACTICE: IDENTIFYING CORRECTLY STATED NURSING DIAGNOSES

Instructions

For the nursing diagnoses listed below, identify those that are correctly stated. NANDA nursing diagnoses should be used for this exercise. For items that are inaccurately stated, correct them using appropriate terminology in the space provided.

1. _____ Skin Integrity, Altered _____
2. _____ Constipation, Perceived _____
3. _____ Fluid Volume, Impaired _____
4. _____ Airway, Obstructed _____
5. _____ Fatigue _____
6. _____ Growth and Development, Altered _____
7. _____ Confusion, Acute _____
8. _____ Incontinence, Urinary and Bowel _____
9. _____ Peripheral Tissue Perfusion, Impaired _____
10. _____ Pneumonia, Risk for _____
11. _____ Hypothermia, Risk for _____
12. _____ Pain, Chronic _____
13. _____ Airway, Compromised _____
14. _____ Body Temperature, Risk for Impaired _____
15. _____ Infection, Risk for _____
16. _____ Infection, Wound _____
17. _____ Breastfeeding, Ineffective _____
18. _____ Thermoregulation, Altered _____
19. _____ Role Performance, Impaired _____
20. _____ Syndrome, Crohn's _____
21. _____ Communication, Altered Verbal _____
22. _____ Abdominal Pain _____
23. _____ Coping, Ineffective _____
24. _____ Self-Concept, Readiness for Enhanced _____
25. _____ Parenting, Risk for Impaired _____
26. _____ Role Strain, Risk for Caregiver _____
27. _____ Family Processes: Alcoholism, Ineffective _____
28. _____ Coping, Defensive _____
29. _____ Injury, Risk for _____
30. _____ Grieving, Anticipatory _____
31. _____ Body Image, Impaired Perceptual _____
32. _____ Anemia, Risk for _____

33. _____ Knowledge Impairment _____

34. _____ Violence, Risk for _____

35. _____ Urinary Incontinence, Urge _____

36. _____ Anxiety _____

37. _____ Lung Cancer _____

38. _____ Stress, Acute _____

39. _____ Fear _____

40. _____ Cardiac Output, Decreased _____

STUDENT PRACTICE: PRACTICING STEP ONE AND STEP TWO OF THE NURSING PROCESS

Instructions

A. *Underline* abnormal signs and symptoms (do not underline complete sentences).
B. Above abnormal data, write O if objective data and S if subjective data.
C. Cluster data into related groups to identify and support each problem.
D. Label actual and risk problems using NANDA nursing diagnoses (include related to, as evidenced by, or risk factors, as appropriate).

General Information

Name: Mr. C. Gonzales
Age: 68 years   **Sex:** Male   **Race:** Hispanic
Admitting Weight: 170 pounds   **Height:** 68 inches
Vital Signs: Blood pressure, 148/92 mm Hg; respirations, 22 breaths/min; pulse, 98 beats/min; temperature, 97.6°F
Client's Perception of Reason for Admission: Short of breath
Allergies: No known allergies (NKA)
Current Medications: Enalapril (Vasotec) 5 mg BID (twice daily); hydrochlorothiazide (HCTZ) 12.5 mg qd (daily)
Admitting Medical Diagnosis: Congestive heart failure
Previous Medical History: Coronary artery disease (CAD), congestive heart failure, hypertension
Family History: Married for 37 years with two grown children and several grandchildren
Social History: Retired from railroad 7 years ago; attends church services weekly; enjoys reading and flying fuel-powered model airplanes

Assessment Data

Oxygenation: Reports difficulty breathing and increased fatigue; sleeps sitting up in a recliner, otherwise, unable to breathe. States he is a nonsmoker. Lung sounds with crackles to bilateral lower lung fields, anterior and posterior; nonproductive cough. Apical pulse 98 beats/min, strong and regular;

radial pulses are equal in strength and quality. Pedal pulses are regular and equal in strength. Denies chest pain. Brisk capillary refill of fingernail beds. Pitting edema assessed to bilateral ankles and feet; rated as two-plus.

Temperature: Afebrile

Nutritional/Fluid: Saline lock inserted in right hand; patent and without erythema (redness) or edema. Reports recent weight gain of 8 pounds over previous 2 weeks. Eats three small meals daily and drinks adequate fluids; no nausea or vomiting.

Gastrointestinal/Elimination: Reports regular bowel movement and urinary elimination patterns. Abdomen is slightly distended, soft, and nontender to palpation. Bowel sounds are present in all four quadrants.

Rest/Sleep: States no energy and is not resting at night. Over previous 2 weeks has had to sleep slightly elevated in his recliner chair or becomes too short of breath. Denies use of sleeping aids and medications.

Pain Avoidance: Denies pain at this time.

Sexuality/Reproduction: Denies difficulties.

Activity: Ambulates without difficulty but becomes short of breath with minimal exertion. States he walks around the block twice weekly.

Additional Data: Patient is alert and oriented; responds appropriately to questions.

Separate data into subjective and objective.

Subjective	Objective

Cluster data into groups of related data to determine problems.

Determine NANDA nursing diagnoses.

_____

_____

_____

_____

_____

_____

_____

_____

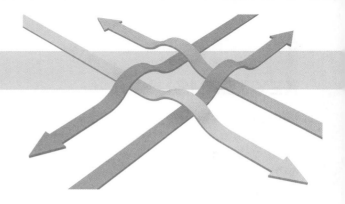

CHAPTER 4

PLANNING

OBJECTIVES

Upon completion of this chapter, the student should be able to:

- ► Define the purposes of the planning phase.
- ► Identify and describe each component of the planning phase.
- ► Distinguish between goals and expected outcomes.
- ► Explain characteristics of nursing interventions and rationales.
- ► Discuss communication and documentation of the care plan.

KEY TERMS

care plan

client centered

dependent nursing
   intervention

discharge planning

expected outcome

goal

independent nursing
   intervention

interdependent nursing
   intervention

long-term goal

measurable

nursing intervention

planning

priorities

rationale

short-term goal

strengths

PLANNING: STEP 3 OF THE NURSING PROCESS

Planning is the third phase of the nursing process. In prior steps, data were collected, analyzed, validated, and organized, and problems and strengths identified and then labeled with the appropriate nursing diagnosis. Nurses then develop a plan of care, which establishes the proposed course of nursing action. The ultimate goal of the planning phase is to promote optimum or an improved level of functioning for the client. Critical elements of planning include:

- Identifying priority problems and interventions
- Setting realistic goals and expected outcomes
- Determining appropriate nursing interventions and recognizing when collaboration is necessary
- Communicating and documenting the proposed care plan

Scientific knowledge and understanding of the holistic needs of the client aid the professional nurse in effective planning. The purpose of this chapter is to explain the above critical components and to stress the importance of effective planning in promoting quality nursing care.

Planning begins as the nurse analyzes the overall data collected during the assessment phase and the client's health care situation. Critical thought and problem solving are necessary skills when planning care. *Priority* problems requiring immediate attention are identified. *Strengths*, the client's *support system*, the health care *facility* itself, and available *resources* are considered as well.

Priority problems are those considered to be more important or life threatening. Priorities are dealt with before less critical problems. For example, Terrence Stewart was involved in an automobile accident and arrived at an emergency care center for treatment. Mr. Stewart began to experience symptoms suspiciously similar to an acute myocardial infarction (heart attack). In addition, he had sustained abrasions (skin scrapes) to his left arm and elbow during the accident. Obviously, the priority in this scenario is providing care to support the client's circulatory system (or cardiac function). The abrasions may be recognized as a problem, but they are less critical.

Strengths include physical, psychological, or personal characteristics. Strengths are thought to *promote* a higher or improved level of functioning. Examples of strengths include:

- Physical: Client has maintained optimal physical condition with exercise or diet.

- Psychological: Client exhibits healthy ways of coping in a crisis.
- Personal: Client is motivated to recover independence; compliance with medical treatment.

Facility refers to the health care delivery facility. The facility must be capable of providing the care necessary for a client. For example, if a client was a resident in a long-term care facility and sustained an injury requiring surgical intervention, this client will most likely require transfer to another facility equipped to provide surgical care. If another client began experiencing chest pain radiating to his left arm, and experienced nausea and shortness of breath (dyspnea), the most appropriate facility would be an emergency department at an acute care facility, not a health clinic.

Resources refer to the ways and means of obtaining health care. For example, is necessary equipment available at the facility? Does the client have transportation to obtain health care? Does the client have health insurance? Can the client afford to purchase medication or equipment prescribed?

Every aspect of the care plan should be *realistic* for both the client and the hospital, facility, or home care setting, depending on client needs.

Purpose and Characteristics of Planning

Planning care must be individualized and realistic for each client. The purpose of planning includes promoting improvement in the client's present state of health or preserving the client's present health status. Planning facilitates adjustment to diminished health, when an improved level of wellness is not possible, or promotes acceptance to the client's deteriorating health. Steps involved in planning include:

- Determining priority problems
- Establishing goals and expected outcomes
- Planning interventions with scientific rationale
- Communicating and documenting the plan of care

DETERMINING PRIORITIES

The first step in planning is determining priorities by recognizing problems that need immediate attention. Obviously, life-threatening situations must be given more urgency than non–life-threatening problems. Consider client preferences by encouraging input. Mutually setting priorities promotes compliance with care and the client's sense of control. Table 4:1 shows common guidelines to assist in priority setting.

Consider *Maslow's hierarchy of needs*. Prioritize according to the basic physiological needs (oxygenation, nutrition, hydration, elimination, body temperature maintenance, and pain avoidance). Generally, basic physiological needs must be met sufficiently, before higher level needs (safe environment, security, love and belonging, and so on) are addressed.

TABLE 4:1 Associating Maslow's Hierarchy of Needs with Priority Problems

Priority 1 Physiological Needs	• Problems interfering with ability to maintain physiological life processes, such as ability to breathe, maintaining a patent airway, maintaining adequate circulation • Problems interfering with homeostatic physiological responses within the body, such as respiration, circulation, hydration, elimination, temperature regulation, nutrition • Problems interfering with ability to be free of offensive stimuli, such as pain, nausea, and other physical irritation
Priority 2 Safety/Security	• Problems interfering with safety and security, such as anxiety, fear, environmental hazards, physical activity deficit, violence towards self or others
Priority 3 Love and Belonging	• Problems interfering with love and belonging, such as sensory-perceptual losses, inability to maintain family and significant other relationships, isolation, loss of a loved one
Priority 4 Self-Esteem	• Problems interfering with self-esteem, such as inability to perform normal daily activities of living, change in physiological structure or function of body or body part
Priority 5 Self-Actualization	• Problems interfering with one's ability for self-actualization, such as positive personal assessment of life events, achieving personal goals

REFLECTION PLANNING AND OUTCOME IDENTIFICATION

After data collection (*assessment phase*), the nurse identified one priority nursing diagnosis of *Deficient Fluid Volume* related to insufficient fluid intake and active fluid loss as evidenced by (defining characteristics) dry mucous membranes, decreased urine output, weakness, reports of frequent diarrhea, and increased urine concentration. Additional nursing diagnoses may be identified during the *diagnosing phase*.

As the *planning phase* begins, the goal and expected outcomes are identified and then nursing interventions are documented to the plan of care.

Client goal:

• Client will demonstrate adequate hydration as evidenced by moist mucous membranes and increased urine output to at least 30 mL per hour within 72 hours.

Client expected outcomes:

- Client will increase PO (by mouth) fluid intake before end of shift.
- Client will report no further episodes of diarrhea within 24 hours.

Nursing interventions:

1. Monitor for the existence of factors causing deficient fluid volume, such as vomiting, diarrhea, or difficulty maintaining oral intake.
2. Monitor total fluid intake and output every 8 hours (or more frequently if unstable).
3. Provide fresh water and oral replacement fluids preferred by the client. Offer frequent drinks, fresh fruits, and fruit juice. Distribute fluids over 24-hour period.
4. Administer antidiarrheal medications as prescribed and appropriate.

Remember, the planning component of the nursing process includes establishing priorities; setting goals and expected outcomes; selecting appropriate nursing interventions; and finally, documenting the plan of care.

Attention to more than one problem may occur simultaneously. For example, the nurse may be performing interventions related to pain reduction and at the same time instructing and encouraging the client about proper use of an incentive spirometer, thus improving the client's oxygenation status.

Finally, priorities may include setting goals and initiating actions to prevent problems from occurring (Table 4:2). Nurses often anticipate potentially serious problems that may arise without nursing intervention.

TABLE 4:2 Prioritizing Nursing Diagnoses with Accompanying Nursing Interventions

Priority	Nursing Diagnosis	Nursing Interventions
High	Risk for Suffocation	• Encourage safety measures • Maintain proper positioning • Suction as needed
Moderate	Risk for Impaired Skin Integrity	• Perform comprehensive skin assessment • Keep skin clean and dry • Provide turning schedule
Low	Ineffective Coping	• Assist to identify problems • Encourage keeping daily journal • Teach client strategies for expressing feelings

Goals and expected outcomes:

- Give direction to the plan of care
- Are used to evaluate the effectiveness of the nursing care plan

ESTABLISHING GOALS AND EXPECTED OUTCOMES

After priority problem identification, setting goals and expected outcomes follows. One overall goal is determined for each nursing diagnosis.

Definition and Components of Goals and Expected Outcomes

The terms *goal*, *outcome*, and *expected outcome* are often used interchangeably. A goal is a general statement indicating the intent or desired change in the client's health status, function, or behavior. An expected outcome is more specific, describing the methods through which the goal will be achieved. Refer to Table 4:3 for goal and expected outcome application examples.

Goals and expected outcomes must be measurable (able to be quantified). The client demonstrates a certain action within a specified time frame. The demonstrated action and time frame are

TABLE 4:3 Application of Goals and Expected Outcomes

Nursing Diagnosis: *Body Image Disturbed*
Goal: Client will demonstrate acceptance of amputation and an ability to adjust to lifestyle change within 6 months.
Expected Outcomes:
• Looks at and touches area of missing body part
• Participates in wound and stump care
• Plans for prosthesis
• Returns to former social involvement
Nursing Diagnosis: *Impaired Gas Exchange*
Goal: Client will maintain a patent airway throughout hospitalization.
Expected Outcomes:
• Verbalizes understanding of oxygen administration and respiratory treatments
• Maintains adequate oxygenation and ventilation
• Remains free of signs of respiratory distress

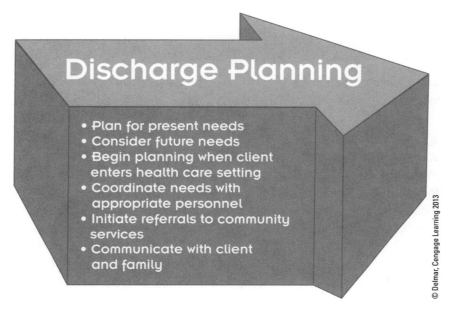

FIGURE 4:1 Goals for Discharge Planning.

the yardsticks that allow the goal or expected outcome to be measured. As interventions planned with goal resolution in mind are carried out, nurses determine how the client responds to each intervention. Favorable responses will most likely lead to attainment of goals and resolution of problems. Goals and expected outcomes provide the health care team with a clear understanding of what is to be accomplished. Goals and expected outcomes are client centered. The client (or part of the client) is expected to achieve a desired outcome.

Goals are constructed by focusing on problem prevention, resolution, or rehabilitation. A short-term goal is a statement identifying a change in behavior that can be achieved fairly quickly, usually within a few hours or days. A long-term goal indicates an objective to be achieved over a longer period, usually over weeks or months. Long-term goals focus on overall greater expectations that may require ongoing health care attention. Discharge planning involves identifying long-term goals, thus promoting continued restorative care and problem resolution through home health, physical therapy, or various other referral sources (Figure 4:1).

After the goal is stated, expected outcomes are identified. Expected outcomes are measurable steps indicating progress toward goal achievement. For each nursing diagnosis and overall goal, there may be several expected outcomes. Both goals and expected outcomes include specific components when appropriately expressed (see Table 4:4 for examples of common mistakes in writing goals). Components include subject, behavior, performance criteria, and time frame.

- The subject identifies the person who will perform the desired behavior or meet the goal. Because goals are client centered, *subject* refers to the client.

TABLE 4:4 Common Mistakes in Writing Goals

Incorrect	Correct
• Focus on the nurse's action when writing the goal	• Goals must be client centered. The *subject* in the goal is the client. For example, *client will demonstrate correct self-administration technique of insulin injection within 48 hours of initial instruction.*
• Statement of unrealistic goal for client. For example, a client with advanced Alzheimer's disease, incontinent of urine, whose care plan goal reads: client will remain continent throughout hospitalization.	• Goals should be realistic. Ask yourself, can the client perform the stated action, thus achieving the goal within the stated time frame? For the incontinent client with advanced Alzheimer's disease, a more appropriate goal might be stated: *client will maintain skin integrity as evidenced by use of continence aids to keep skin dry throughout shift.*
• Goal lacks time frame	• The time frame indicates *when* the goal should be achieved. Otherwise, determination of the client's success or failure in achieving the desired result cannot be evaluated. Appropriately stated goals require four components: subject (*the client*), behavior (*will maintain*), criteria of performance (*skin integrity*), and time frame (*throughout shift*). A fifth component, conditions, is optional. In the example above, *use of continence aids to keep skin dry,* is the condition.
• More than one task or behavior to be accomplished in one goal statement. For example, client will demonstrate a tolerable level of discomfort and will identify at least two alternative measures to reduce pain level within 8 hours.	• Only one behavior should be specified for each goal. Goals will be more explicit and directly measurable.

• Behavior describes *what* the client will do to achieve the goal (see Table 4:5 for examples of measurable verbs). Behavior can be felt, heard, seen, or measured. For example:

  • Will verbalize
  • Will ambulate
  • Will report
  • Will eat
  • Will demonstrate

TABLE 4:5 Measurable Verbs

Identify	Describe	Perform	Relate
State	List	Verbalize	Hold
Demonstrate	Share	Express	Sit
Exercise	Communicate	Stand	Discuss
Cough	Walk	Describe	Reestablish

- The criteria of performance refer to the standards indicating the level of behavior, such as how long, how far, or how much. Criteria of performance may include a time limit, amount of activity, or description of the behavior to be followed.

Examples include:

- Understanding of medication regimen
- Length of the hall
- Decrease in pain level of 4 or less
- 75% of meal
- Decreased blood pressure within 48 hours

- Conditions, *an optional component*, refer to the aid or conditions that facilitate the performance. Conditions may provide clarity. They include experiences the client is expected to have before performing the behavior. For example:

- With the assistance of physical therapy
- With the administration of analgesics
- With the assistance of family
- With the use of medication and diet therapy

- The time frame refers to when the behavior should be accomplished. For example:

- Within 48 hours
- By third postoperative day
- Within 45 minutes
- In 24 hours
- Within 3 weeks of medication therapy

WRITING GOAL AND OUTCOME STATEMENTS

The following are examples of goals stated correctly:

- Client will ambulate assisted by physical therapy to nurse's station and back to room twice daily.
- Client will verbalize understanding of medication regimen prior to discharge.
- Client's skin will demonstrate no evidence of breakdown throughout hospitalization.
- Ms. James will lose 2.5 pounds within 3 weeks by using prescribed American Heart Association diet plan.

- Client will ambulate unassisted with crutches by discharge.
- Client will demonstrate correct injection technique by September 18.

Nursing Interventions Classification (NIC) and Nursing Outcomes Classification (NOC) Defined

The University of Iowa (Iowa Intervention Project) developed the nomenclature of nursing interventions known as *Nursing Interventions Classifications* (NIC), directed toward health promotion and illness management. NIC continues to refine the standardized language that describes nursing interventions performed in all practice settings. NIC is a method for linking nursing interventions to diagnoses and client outcomes. Each intervention is labeled, defined, and lists activities the nurse performs while carrying out the intervention (University of Iowa [n.d.]).

With nursing communities placing greater interest on nursing outcomes, nurse researchers at the University of Iowa have further developed classifications, *Nursing Outcomes Classification* (NOC), of client outcomes. According to the University of Iowa, an outcome is a measurable individual, family or community state, behavior, or perception that is measured along a continuum and is responsive to nursing interventions. NOC continues to be refined for measuring effects of nursing practice. Nursing researchers are involved in observing, measuring, and studying client outcomes that indicate the quality of effectiveness on the nursing interventions provided.

STUDENT PRACTICE: WRITING GOALS

Instructions

For each nursing diagnosis write an appropriate goal. (Remember goal components.)

1. Joe Johnson has experienced intermittent nausea for approximately 6 months because of a possible gastric ulcer. He states, "I know I should eat, but when I eat, I hurt." He has lost 28 pounds since his last annual checkup and weighs less than is ideal for his height. His nurse identifies the nursing diagnosis: *Imbalanced Nutrition: Less Than Body Requirements*; R/T: inability to ingest nutrients as a result of biological factors; AEB: reported food intake less than recommended daily allowance; weight loss of 28 pounds over the past year.

_____

_____

2. Hannah Miller, a neonate, is experiencing a fluctuation in her body temperature from normal to below normal range. Her nurse discovers that Hannah's mother does not keep her covered appropriately. The nurse identifies the nursing diagnosis: *Risk for Hypothermia*; risk factors: exposure to cool environment, inadequate clothing, extremes of age (newborn).

_____

_____

3. Mr. Cooper had abdominal surgery 1 day ago. He has a medical history of diabetes mellitus and must take morning and evening insulin subcutaneously. His nurse identifies the nursing diagnosis: *Risk for Infection*; R/T: inadequate primary defenses (surgical incision/broken skin), increased environmental exposure, chronic disease, invasive procedures.

_____

_____

4. Mr. Sanders states he has been traveling out of the country. Since his return last week, he has been experiencing abdominal cramping and several liquid stools. The nursing diagnosis identified is *Diarrhea*; R/T: gastrointestinal disorder; AEB: abdominal cramping, increased frequency of defecation, liquid stools.

_____

_____

5. Mrs. O'Conner was admitted to the hospital diagnosed with pneumonia. Assessment reveals bilateral wheezes in the midanterior lung fields and mild dyspnea. The nurse observes Mrs. O'Conner coughing up copious amounts of thick, yellow sputum. The nursing diagnosis is identified as *Ineffective Airway Clearance*; R/T: tracheobronchial infection; AEB: abnormal breath sounds (wheezes), productive cough, dyspnea.

_____

_____

Nursing Tip

Planning is prioritizing the identified nursing diagnoses, writing client-centered goals and expected outcomes, developing specific nursing interventions, and recording the plan of care.

PLANNING NURSING INTERVENTIONS

After prioritizing problems and setting goals, nurses use problem-solving and decision-making skills in determining which actions will aid in problem resolution. **Nursing interventions** are specified activities executed by the nursing team that benefit the client in a predictable manner.

Characteristics of Nursing Interventions

Nursing interventions are activities or actions planned by the nurse to produce problem resolution, problem reduction, or prevention of risk problems. Nursing interventions may be planned to assist the client accept his or her present state of health or illness. Nursing interventions specify activities to execute. They focus on the etiology of the problem and may determine when activities are to be carried out, how often, and the duration of each activity.

Nursing interventions are communicated to other nurses involved in the client's treatment by verbal or written report and through documentation of the plan, which promotes continuity of care.

Nursing Tip

Nursing interventions involve:

- *Assisting with activities of daily living (ADLs)*
- *Delivering skilled therapeutic interventions*
- *Discharge planning*
- *Monitoring response to medical and nursing care*
- *Supervising and coordinating nursing personnel*
- *Teaching the client*

Guidelines for Selecting Nursing Interventions

Appropriate interventions are selected using guiding principles provided by official nurse regulating organizations, such as nurse practice act and state boards of nursing standards. Nurses must practice within the legal realm of nursing guidelines and boundaries. Furthermore, interventions must be realistic for the client and nurse, as well as for the facility. Nurses consider the client's values and beliefs and the consequences and risks of each intervention.

Classification of Nursing Interventions

Nursing interventions are classified according to three categories:

- Independent
- Interdependent
- Dependent

Independent nursing interventions are nursing actions initiated by the nurse not requiring direction or an order from another health care professional. They are actions regulated by state boards of nursing and nurse practice acts, which allow nurses to independently intervene depending on client needs. Interventions may support ADLs, health education, health promotion, and counseling. For example, the environment may be managed by nurses to establish and maintain a safe, therapeutic environment, promote rest, reduce noise, maintain cleanliness, or manage environmental temperature.

Interdependent nursing interventions are actions developed in consultation or collaboration with other health care professionals to gain another's viewpoint in determining an intervention most beneficial for the client. An example is discussion of the client in an interdisciplinary conference for discharge planning attended by the primary nurse or supervisor, home health care nurse, social worker, physical therapist, and dietician.

Nurses may consult with specialists when the problem cannot be resolved using their personal knowledge or skills. Specialists may be consulted to determine the best method for nursing diagnosis resolution, for example, consulting a dietician regarding a special diet.

Dependent nursing interventions are actions requiring an order from a physician or another health care professional, such as a request for physician-prescribed medication orders. Likewise, nurses may question a previously written order based on knowledge of current client status or change in the client's condition, requesting clarification or new orders.

Where Do Nursing Interventions Originate?

Interventions may originate from written or verbal physician orders. The physician relies on the nurse's judgment and ability to carry out orders in a safe, effective manner. Nursing interventions may be written to complement the physician-prescribed treatments (see Table 4:6).

Nursing interventions may result from such client needs as health-related teaching, counseling, or referrals to other health care professionals. Interventions may involve specific nursing treatments or collection of ongoing assessment data related to client status. Other interventions may evolve from measures to take during basic care, such as suctioning, repositioning, assisting with nutrition, providing hygiene measures, assisting with ADLs, providing emotional support, or maintaining range of motion.

Example:
Nursing diagnosis: *Activity intolerance*; R/T: bed rest, generalized weakness; AEB: verbalization of overwhelming lack of energy, dyspnea on exertion while performing activities of daily living.

Goal: *Client will verbalize improved level of energy when carrying out activities of daily living within 1 week.*

1. Assess ability to perform ADLs.
2. Evaluate adequacy of nutrition and sleep.
3. Schedule periods of uninterrupted time for client to rest throughout the day.
4. Assist client with activities of daily living as necessary. Promote and encourage ADL independence without causing exhaustion.

TABLE 4:6 Types of Nursing Orders

Type	Description	Example
Health promotion	Encouraging behaviors leading to a higher level of wellness	• Reinforce the importance of a daily exercise regimen. • Encourage client to begin keeping a journal of daily exercises performed.
Observation/monitoring patient status	Monitoring client for potential complications and response to performed nursing interventions	• Encourage client to report increasing pain level before it becomes severe. • Monitor blood pressure prior to administering antihypertensive medications as ordered by provider.
Prevention	Reducing risk factors or preventing complications	• Encourage client to use incentive spirometer every 2 hours and monitor performance. • Advise client and family members in proper handwashing method.
Treatment	Teaching, referrals, or performing physical care necessary in the treatment of an existing problem	• Teach client proper technique for diabetic foot care. • Request referral for dietary consult.

Interventions are prioritized according to the order in which they will be implemented or carried out. Several interventions should be identified for each goal.

Scientific Rationales

As previously explained, interventions are selected based on an understanding of scientific principles and psychosocial or developmental theories. Understanding of the human body and mind allows for certain expected responses when interventions are carried out. Rationales are the underlying reasons for which the intervention was chosen. When interventions are chosen, nursing students should identify and provide scientific rationale for each intervention. This action aids in further understanding of the theoretical and scientific knowledge of nursing.

Example:

The nurse is caring for a client medically diagnosed with emphysema who refuses to quit smoking cigarettes.

Nursing diagnosis: *Noncompliance* (therapeutic regimen)

R/T: client value system, health belief

AEB: failure to adhere to health recommendations, evidence of exacerbation of symptoms

Goal: *Client will communicate an understanding of disease process and treatment within 48 hours.*

Nursing Intervention: Collaborate with client to implement a plan for smoking cessation.

Rationale: *Active participation in decision making about therapeutic regimen may increase compliance.*

Scientific research has provided proof that a client who participates in health care decision making is more likely to be compliant. These data may be located in research articles, fundamental or foundation textbooks, nursing journals, and other resources. Identify the *key subject* or *term*, such as decision making or compliance, and then locate the rationale in one of the resources or references.

Nursing Tip

Determine key words in interventions and diagnoses, such as postsurgery and hypoxia. Rationales for these are found in medical-surgical textbook chapters relating to any client undergoing surgery for any reason. Hypoxia is a postoperative complication for which the nurse must monitor.

Example:

For the client who had orthopedic surgery:

Nursing intervention: Monitor airway and respiratory pattern every 2 hours for initial 8 to 12 hours or until stable.

Rationale: *Most anesthetic agents depress respiratory rate and depth, thus interfering with oxygenation of the blood.*

Side effects and adverse effects of anesthetic agents are found in resources, such as medical-surgical textbooks discussing the care of surgical clients.

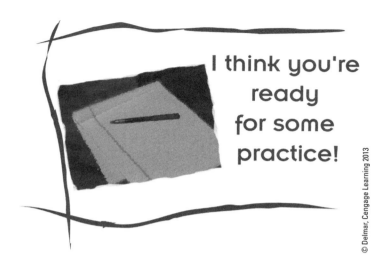

I think you're
ready
for some
practice!

© Delmar, Cengage Learning 2013

STUDENT PRACTICE: SCIENTIFIC RATIONALES

Instructions

Determine scientific rationales for each nursing intervention below.

Nursing diagnosis: *Activity intolerance*; R/T: bed rest, generalized weakness; AEB: verbalization of overwhelming lack of energy, dyspnea on exertion while performing ADLs

Goal: *Client will verbalize improved level of energy when carrying out ADLs within 1 week.*

Nursing Interventions:

1. Assess ability to perform ADLs. _____

   _____

   _____

2. Determine the cause of activity intolerance and determine if the cause is physical or motivational.

   _____

   _____

3. Encourage client to be out of bed. Increase activity gradually. _____

   _____

   _____

4. Allow client sufficient time to carry out ADLs and give adequate rest periods between activities. Provide assistance as necessary. _____

   _____

   _____

COMMUNICATING AND DOCUMENTING THE CARE PLAN

The client's plan of care is documented according to hospital policy and becomes part of the client's permanent medical record. The care plan is shared with other members of the health care team who are actively caring for the client. The plan may be reviewed by the oncoming nurse or communicated in part during report.

KEY CONCEPTS

- Planning is the third phase in the nursing process. Critical elements of planning include identifying priority problems and interventions, setting realistic goals and expected outcomes, determining nursing interventions and rationales for each intervention, and finally, communication and documentation of the care plan.
- Establishing priorities may be guided by factors such as endangerment to life, client preferences, and Maslow's hierarchy of needs.
- The care plan is realistic and practical. It considers the client's values, beliefs, and strengths, as well as physical and psychological health.
- Planning individualized care for the client may promote improvement of health, preserve the client's present state of health, help the client to adjust to diminished or a decreasing level of health, or assist the client in accepting deteriorating health.
- A goal indicates the desired change in the client's health status. Goals are client centered and give direction to the care plan. Goals are constructed by focusing on problem prevention, resolution, or rehabilitation. Components of a goal statement include the subject, behavior, criteria of performance, conditions, and time frame.
- Expected outcomes are more specific than goals and describe the methods through which the goal is achieved.
- Goals and expected outcomes are used to measure the success of the care plan. Goals and expected outcomes are stated in a manner that makes them measurable.
- Nursing interventions are actions to be carried out by the nurse and are expected to benefit the client in a predictable manner. Interventions are developed to meet goal objectives and therefore aid in problem resolution.
- Nursing interventions are selected based on the nurse's understanding of scientific principles and psychological or developmental theories. Rationales are the underlying scientific reason for which the intervention was chosen.
- The nursing care plan is a formal written document that becomes part of the client's permanent medical record.
- Documentation and communication of the plan promotes continuity of care.

STUDENT PRACTICE: PLANNING AND OUTCOME IDENTIFICATION

Instructions

Using the scenario from Chapter 3, Mr. C. Gonzales, whose medical diagnosis is congestive heart failure (CHF):

1. Complete all steps involved in planning and outcome identification. (See chart, Figure 4:2.)
2. Identify two or three priority problems. For each problem, determine one nursing diagnosis statement (label, R/T, and AEB), one goal, and three interventions with scientific rationale.

Name: _____ Date: _____

Care plan documentation form: For each nursing diagnosis, include R/T, AEB, or risk factors (for risk nursing diagnosis); one goal/expected outcome per nursing diagnosis; and at least three nursing interventions with scientific rationale for each nursing intervention. Evaluate goal/expected outcome when appropriate (one evaluative statement).

Nursing Diagnosis (with R/T + AEB)

_____

_____

Goal

_____

_____

Nursing Interventions (with *Scientific Rationale*)

1. _____

_____

_____

2. _____

_____

_____

3. _____

_____

_____

Evaluation

_____

_____

FIGURE 4:2 Care Plan Documentation Form.

CHAPTER 5

IMPLEMENTATION

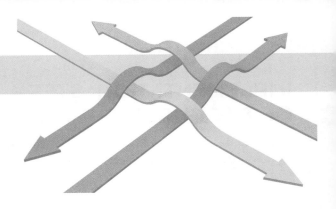

OBJECTIVES

Upon completion of this chapter, the student should be able to:

▶ Discuss the purpose of the implementation phase of the nursing process.

▶ Describe ways in which the care plan is implemented.

▶ Identify the relationship between assessment and implementation.

▶ Discuss communication and documentation of client response to interventions as they are implemented.

▶ Describe key components of recording and reporting, including data to document on the client's chart and data to report to oncoming personnel.

▶ Discuss confidentiality and the client's right to privacy.

KEY TERMS

confidentiality
documentation
focus charting

implementation
Kardex
narrative charting

PIE charting
reporting

IMPLEMENTATION: STEP 4 OF THE NURSING PROCESS

Implementation is the fourth phase of the nursing process. During this phase, activities such as executing nursing interventions, performing an ongoing assessment of the client, and determining the client's response to executed interventions are observed, communicated, and documented. As with all prior steps of the nursing process, nurses demonstrate knowledge and understanding of physical and social sciences and apply analytical skills and deliberate thought processes to interpret client responses to interventions. Nurses participate in ongoing assessment as implementation takes place. This chapter discusses the purpose and characteristics of implementation, guidelines for reporting and recording, and the client's right to privacy and confidentiality.

Nursing Tip

Nursing implementation activities include identifying priority intervention; ongoing assessment before, during, and after interventions are performed; and documenting interventions and client responses.

Characteristics of Implementation

The implementation phase is directed at meeting the client's needs through execution of interventions and evaluation of client response. These actions ultimately result in health promotion, prevention of illness, or restoration of health. The client is encouraged to provide input in care planning and priority identification, thus promoting compliance and giving the client a sense of control.

Nursing professionals monitor the client's response to treatment and therapies through means of physical assessment and communication with the client. Nurses analyze the client's response. Evaluation may include additional investigation, such as reviewing laboratory results, progress notes, and collaborating with the physician and other nurses involved in the client's care. Accurate reporting and recording of all pertinent data are necessary.

REFLECTION IMPLEMENTATION

The nurse is providing care for an 83-year-old man who recently was diagnosed with a cerebro-vascular accident (stroke). The nursing process was initiated after admission to the floor, and one priority nursing diagnosis was determined to be *Impaired Swallowing* related to neuromus-cular impairment and decreased or absent gag reflex as evidence by (defining characteristics) abnormality in oral phase of swallow study, choking, coughing before swallowing, and inability to clear oral cavity.

The overall goal for this client is that he will remain free from aspiration throughout hospitalization.

The nurse goes to the client's hospital room to carry out one of the nursing interventions included in the client's plan of care, which is to observe and assist with meals. *Before* attempt-ing to assist with his meal, the nurse will assess the client. Is he awake, alert, and able to follow directions? Is he in the correct anatomical position, sitting upright at 90 degrees? Is he able to swallow liquids? Additional safety precautions will be followed as the nurse attempts to assist with the client's meal and prevent aspiration.

The nurse completes her initial assessment and then begins the intervention. Ongoing assessment continues as she carries out the nursing intervention, carefully observing, giving him instructions, providing adequate time, and checking his oral cavity for proper emptying.

After the intervention is completed, the nurse documents data determined during the cli-ent's initial assessment, how the client responded to the intervention, and the client's current status.

Remember, assessment is a continuous process. As nursing interventions are carried out, the nurse is assessing the client before, during, and after each intervention is carried out.

DOCUMENTATION

Several factors are considered for documentation to be effective. Documentation is the process of preparing a record reflecting the assessment data and both the client's health status and response to care. Depending on the facility, various formats may be used. Guidelines for documentation include the following:

- Ensure that you have the correct client record or chart and that the client's name and identifying information are on every page of the record.
- Document as soon as the client encounter is concluded to ensure accurate recall of data (follow institutional guidelines on frequency of charting).
- Date and time each entry.
- Sign each entry with your full legal name and with your professional credentials or per your institutional policy.

- Do not leave space between entries.
- If an error is made while documenting, use a single line to cross out the error and then date, time, and sign the correction (check institutional policy); avoid erasing, crossing out, or using correction fluid.
- Never change another person's entry even if it is incorrect.
- Use quotation marks to indicate direct client responses (e.g., "I feel lousy").
- Document in chronological order (if chronological order is not used, state why).
- Write legibly.
- Use a permanent ink pen (black is usually preferable because of its ability to photocopy well).
- Document in a complete but concise manner by using phrases and abbreviations as appropriate.
- Document all telephone calls that you make or receive that are related to a client's case.

(Adapted from Estes, M.E.Z. [2010]. *Health assessment and physical examination* [4th ed.]. Clifton Park, NY: Delmar Cengage Learning.)

Assessment Specific Documentation Guidelines

- Record all data that contribute directly to the assessment (e.g., positive assessment findings and pertinent negatives).
- Document any parts of the assessment that are omitted or refused by the client.
- Avoid using judgmental language such as "good," "poor," "bad," "normal," "abnormal," "decreased," "appears to be," and "seems."
- Avoid evaluative statements (e.g., "client is uncooperative," "client is lazy"); cite instead specific statements or actions that you observe (e.g., "client said, 'I hate this place' and kicked trash receptacle").
- State time intervals precisely (e.g., "every 4 hours," "bid," instead of "seldom," "occasionally").
- Do not make relative statements about findings (e.g., "mass the size of an egg"); use specific measurements (e.g., "mass 3 cm × 5 cm").
- Draw pictures when appropriate (e.g., location of scar, masses, skin lesion, decubitus, deep tendon reflex).
- Refer to findings using anatomical landmarks (e.g., left upper quadrant [of abdomen], left lower lobe [of lung], midclavicular line).
- Use the face of the clock to describe findings that are in a circular pattern (e.g., breast, tympanic membrane, rectum, vagina).
- Document any change in the client's condition during a visit or from previous visits.
- Describe what you observed, not what you did.

(Adapted from Estes, M.E.Z. [2010]. *Health assessment and physical examination* [4th ed.]. Clifton Park, NY: Delmar Cengage Learning.)

Figure 5:1 compares examples of correctly and incorrectly documented data in a 24-hour record.

SEE CARE PLAN
NURSING DIAGNOSIS:

Date	Time	Progress Notes
X/XX/XX	0840	A~~~~ completed by nurses aid.----------CmnUSA21
	0930	16F Foley cath inserted, s~~~~ que. 450cc clear yellow urine out.
	1100	Husband at bedside. Seems to be mad at wife. J.Minton RN
	1340	Pt. To X-ray via ~~stretcher~~ wheelchair.

Do not leave blank lines between entries.

Write legibly. Sign each entry with name and credentials.

Do not leave blank spaces after entry.

When an error is made, draw one line through entry. Write 'incorrect entry' and initial.

SEE CARE PLAN
NURSING DIAGNOSIS:

Date	Time	Progress Notes
X/XX/XX	0700	Received pt. Sitting on bedside chair. Respirations, even, un-labored. Skin warm, dry. No distress noted.-J.Minton RN
	0845	Breakfast served, family at bedside. Denies dyspnea or----chest pain at this time, however, using ~~accessory muscles~~ incorrect entry - JH accessory muscles to breath, at rest.----J. Minton RN

FIGURE 5:1 Examples of incorrect and correct documentation.

Nursing Tip

Effective documentation requires:

- *Use of a common vocabulary*
- *Legibility and neatness*
- *Use of only authorized abbreviations and symbols*
- *Factual and timesequenced organization*
- *Accurately including any errors that occurred*
- *Following facility protocol*

Documentation Methods

Depending on your facility, many different systems may be utilized for documentation purposes: electronic medical records (EMR), narrative, PIE (problem-intervention-evaluation), focus, and others. Always be familiar with your facility's documentation policies and procedures and document within those guidelines.

Narrative Charting

Narrative charting refers to a traditional, sequential, documentation system. The nurse describes the client's status, physical assessment, interventions and treatments, and the client's response to treatments. Narrative charting has been replaced in many institutions because:

- The flow of care is disorganized.
- It fails to reflect the nursing process.
- It is time consuming.
- Specific information is difficult to retrieve.

Be specific and descriptive when documenting narrative notes. See the acronym CHARTING in Table 5:1 for data to include.

PIE Charting

PIE (problem-intervention-evaluation) charting organizes information according to problems the client is experiencing, interventions performed, and evaluation of client response. Assessment flow sheets and progress notes are maintained on a daily basis. Initial assessment determines problems, labels them as nursing diagnoses, and numbers them for future reference. For example, when the nurse documents data regarding problem one, the entry notation begins with *P #1*. For interventions performed in relation to problem one, the entry notation begins with *I-P #1* followed by the entry. When the nurse evaluates the response to an intervention for problem one, the entry

TABLE 5:1 Documentation to Include While Charting

Condition: current condition of the client, physically, emotionally; condition of wounds/dressings; change in condition of the client

Happenings: abnormal or variations from usual routine; visits from family, physician, discharge instructions

Additions: changes to the care plan; abnormal laboratory values

Response: to interventions carried out, reactions or response to medications administered, reports received or given to other personnel

Treatments, transfers, transport to other departments

Invasive procedures performed

Notes: refers to narrative notes when the flow sheet is not enough

Good job!

SEE CARE PLAN
NURSING DIAGNOSIS:

DATE	TIME	NOTES
XX/XX/XXXX	13.30	P#1 = Complaints of acute pain to right lower quadrant
		abdomen. Rates as "7" on scale of 1 to 10.
		I P#1 = adm. Analgesics as prescribed. Monitor quality,
		location, intensity, & frequency. Document. Encourage
		diversional activities, such as music, focus breathing
		reading, etc. Advise to request analgesic prior to pain
		Becoming intense————————————W.Seaback RN
		EP#1 = pain resolves. Client requests analgesics when
		pain level "4" or less on scale of 1 to 10. Participates
		in diversional activities. VS remain within normal limits.
		Client reports further symptoms.———— W.Seaback RN
XX/XX/XXXX	13.30	P#2 = Risk for Infection RT surgical incision
		I P#2 = sterile wound care qd, as per MD orders.
		Monitor wound for signs of redness, edema, drainage,
		odor, approximation. Monitor for temp elevation. Adm.
		Antibiotics as ordered.——————————W.Seaback RN
		EP#2 = incision heals without evidence of infection. No
		temp elevation.———————————————W.Seaback RN

© Delmar, Cengage Learning 2013

FIGURE 5:2 PIE charting example.

notation begins with *E-P #1* followed by the evaluation entry, and so on. Figure 5:2 shows an example of PIE documentation.

FOCUS Charting

The focus charting system involves documentation of three categories: *data, action,* and *response,* or DAR. Figure 5:3 shows an example of a focus charting system. The D or *data* category is the focus of the entry. Each focus may include specific identified problems stated as nursing diagnoses or may identify the topic of the entry. Examples of data may include:

- A nursing diagnosis, such as *Impaired Mobility*
- Subjective or objective data, such as description of a wound or abdominal pain
- Client behavior, such as ability to perform ADLs
- Change in the client's condition, such as labored respiration or experiencing chest pain
- A significant event, such as debridement of a wound
- A special need, such as referral to home health care service

The A or *action* category includes nursing actions based on assessment of the client's condition. An example is administering an analgesic in response to the client's subjective statement of severe pain. The action entry includes the executed intervention. It may also include changes to the care plan deemed necessary, resulting from the nurse's assessment.

SEE CARE PLAN
NURSING DIAGNOSIS:

Date	Time	Focus	Progress Notes
XX/XX/XXXX	0945	Consti-	D: Pt states no BM for 4 days. Abdominal
		pation	cramping. Bowel sounds hypoactive X 4 quads
	1015		A: administered 1000 cc warm, tap-water
			enema. Advised to hold as long as possible.
	1055		A: assisted to bedside commode. Call bell
			within reach.----------------W.Seaback RN
	1100		R: Client expelled large amount of dark,
			brown, formed stool, large amount of liquid
			and flatus.---------------W.Seaback RN
	1130		A: assisted into bed. Provided perineal care.
			D: excoriation noted to perineal area. Skin
			barrier applied. -------------W.Seaback RN
	1300	Nutri-	D: client ate 75% of soft mechanical diet.
		tion	No nausea at this time.------W.Seaback RN

© Delmar, Cengage Learning 2013

FIGURE 5:3 FOCUS charting example.

The *response* category (R) describes the client's response to nursing care, medical care, or specific interventions. In the example of administering an analgesic for severe pain, the response entry might include a statement noting severe pain was resolved.

Computerized Documentation

Many health care organizations have implemented computerized documentation in response to the large demand for clinical, administrative, and regulatory information. Health care facilities work in collaboration with producers of computer software to design medical record documents that complement existing documentation systems. There are advantages and disadvantages to computerized documentation.

Advantages Include

- Enhances the systematic approach to client care through standardized protocols, teaching documents, management, and communication.
- Computers are cost-effective and increase the quality of documentation.
- Saves documentation time. Data entry needs to be done only once; the system avoids duplication of entries.
- Increases legibility and accuracy. The program prompts the nurse for information, making the charting more complete, thorough, concise, and organized.
- Provides clear, decisive, and concise key words. Standardized nursing terminology provides usage of consistent key words. Nurses may select choices on a screen that automatically builds a comprehensive record of an event.
- Facilitates statistical analysis of data.

- Enhances critical thinking and decision making by providing access to other data, such as laboratory results that can be correlated with the nurses' assessment data.
- Supports multidisciplinary networking. Information is quickly coordinated and integrated by other departments and all departments have access to data.

Disadvantages Include

- Computer and software may limit the number of terminals at nursing stations.
- Cost of installation.
- Processing speed may be slower at peak usage times.
- Sudden unexpected failure of the computer or software and downtime for routine servicing.

Kardex

A Kardex may or may not be used at a particular health care facility. The Kardex is a condensed reference tool that includes basic client care information. The Kardex is often used during change-of-shift reports, providing cues regarding pertinent information to discuss or relay. The Kardex may also be utilized as a quick reference throughout the shift.

When a client is admitted onto the nursing unit, data from the physician's admitting orders are generally penciled onto the card. As new physician orders are received, the Kardex is updated to reflect the change.

Information contained on the Kardex may vary in different facilities; however, the Kardex often includes data such as:

- Client data: name, age, sex, height, and weight
- Emergency data: name of contact person, relationship, address, and telephone number
- Daily diagnostic examinations, scheduled examinations, or surgery
- Medical diagnoses: admitting and history
- Nursing diagnoses: by priority
- Medical orders: diet, DNR (do not resuscitate) status, isolation, restraints, invasive procedures, vital sign parameters, activity, treatments, such as sitz bath or antiembolytic stockings
- Special therapies: respiratory therapy, physical therapy, and/or occupational therapy
- Routine medications including dosage amounts, times, intravenous solutions and medication, and as-needed medications

REPORTING

Reporting includes verbal communication of facts regarding the client's health status and ongoing care provided. When a report is given, the nurse summarizes the current critical information to facilitate continuity of care. Thought should be given to what data are necessary to report. Table 5:2 identifies an acronym, RECEIVE, with examples of data to include while reporting. Verbal reports may be required in a variety of situations, such as reporting to:

- Oncoming shift personnel with summary reports or walking rounds
- A receiving unit or facility via telephone when the client is transferred or discharged
- A superior who is in charge or the health care provider

TABLE 5:2 Information to Include in a Verbal Report

Reporting: facts, not opinions. Report objectively and accurately; be concise and complete.

Essential information: about the client, such as name, age, sex, admission medical diagnosis, and pertinent history data

Condition: current condition, such as diet, nothing by mouth (NPO), do not resuscitate (DNR) status, response to administered medication, Foley catheter, IV solution and site, orientation, prescribed activity level, fluid restriction, assistance needed by client, current teaching and client response.

Extra medications: such as last prn (as needed) pain medication administered, preoperative medications on call or administered, medications to be given dependent on laboratory values. For example, "Give 20 mEq KCl for potassium <3.0."

Identify priorities: relating to care, upcoming procedures, recurring laboratory tests, diagnostic tests completed, and results if known. Identify activities completed and those to be completed.

Values: such as last blood glucose level, vital sign parameters, abnormal vital signs, intake and output amounts.

Exceptional report given!

Nursing Tip

Always maintain client **confidentiality.** *What does this term mean to you?*

CONFIDENTIALITY

Information obtained from or about the client is considered to be *privileged* and, in most cases, cannot be disclosed to a third party. Clients have a legal and ethical right to privacy. As a student or practicing nurse, you have a legal and ethical responsibility for protecting client confidentiality. Be familiar with HIPAA regulations. The Health Insurance Portability and Accountability Act of 1996 provides protection for personal health information held by covered entities, such as client care data found on client care records, and gives clients an array of rights with respect to that information. The HIPAA privacy rule is balanced so that it permits the disclosure to personal health information needed for client care. Federal and state laws ensure no one will reveal the client's confidential information without permission. Nurses should not disclose information about the client's status to other clients or staff not involved in the client's care. Nurses should not discuss any client's condition in inappropriate settings, such as the cafeteria or elevator. Nurses must obtain the client's permission before disclosing any information regarding the client, going through the client's personal belongings, performing procedures, and photographing the client.

KEY CONCEPTS

- Implementation is the fourth step in the nursing process. During implementation, nursing interventions are executed, and the client's response is observed, communicated, and documented.
- As nurses interact with the client, assessment continues throughout each phase of the nursing process. New data are collected as the client responds to treatment, therapies, and nursing interventions.
- Client responses are reported to other health care professionals involved in the client's care and recorded in the 24-hour client care record (nurse's notes).
- Nurses are ethically and legally obligated to protect client confidentiality and privacy.

STUDENT PRACTICE: DOCUMENTATION

Instructions

Read the brief vignette below.

A. Rewrite data in *narrative* documentation format.
B. Rewrite data in *focus* documentation format.

Complete sentences are not necessary.

Vignette: This morning when day shift began, Mr. James was lying in bed with his eyes closed. When the nurse touched his arm, his skin was warm and dry. Mr. James's respirations were even and unlabored. He did not appear to be in any distress. Report was completed at 0715. When breakfast was served, around 0815, he was watching television. Mr. James complained of muscle spasms to his right lower calf (client recently fractured right tibia). Capillary refill to his right great toe is less than 2 seconds. Feet are warm to touch and he moves them without difficulty. Skin condition around the cast edges is intact and without evidence of skin breakdown. Dr. Martin was called on the telephone at 0830 to advise of muscle spasms and to request new orders. Dr. Martin was in to see the client at 0955. He wrote an order for Mr. James to receive a new medication to reduce muscle spasms. Discharge orders were written. Mr. James states his wife will arrive within the hour for completion of discharge.

A: Narrative Documentation:

Date	Time	

B: Focus Documentation:

Date	Time	Focus	

STUDENT PRACTICE: CHANGE-OF-SHIFT REPORT

Instructions

Locate Student Practice case scenario for client Mr. C. Gonzales in Chapter 3. Using the data provided, determine information that would be necessary to report during change of shift.

_____

_____

_____

_____

_____

_____

_____

_____

_____

_____

_____

_____

_____

_____

_____

CHAPTER 6

EVALUATION

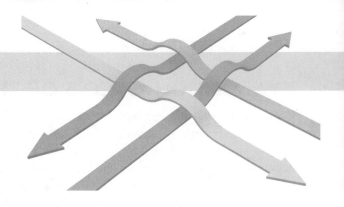

OBJECTIVES

Upon completion of this chapter, the student should be able to:

► Discuss the purpose of evaluation related to the nursing process.

► Identify characteristics of the evaluation phase and how to document evaluation.

► Discuss the relationship between assessment and evaluation.

► Identify how to evaluate effective goal achievement.

► Discuss when it is necessary to modify, revise, or discontinue portions of the care plan.

KEY TERMS

discontinue
evaluation

evaluative statement
goal attainment

modification
revision

EVALUATION: STEP 5 OF THE NURSING PROCESS

Evaluation is the fifth phase of the nursing process. This step takes a critical look at the *results* of implemented nursing interventions. Although evaluation is the final step described in the nursing process, it is interwoven throughout all other steps. Evaluation involves critical analysis of the plan, beginning with initial data collection and continuing through implementation (Figure 6:1). Similar to assessment, evaluation is continuous and ongoing. Interventions and client responses are evaluated with questions. For example: Is the client progressing toward goal resolution? Have goals been met? Is this portion of the plan complete and no longer a problem for the client? Have goals been partially met or not met? When the client is not progressing as expected, answers are sought to determine why.

This chapter describes the purpose, characteristics, components, and methods for evaluation. The chapter also discusses evaluation of goal achievement, as well as determination of how and when to revise, modify, or discontinue the care plan.

Nursing Tip

Degrees of goal attainment include the goal is met, partially met, or not met.

Evaluation Purpose

The purpose of the evaluation phase is to gauge the effectiveness of nursing care and the quality of care provided. Nurses evaluate client responses to determine if the care plan is working or how well the care plan is working and whether the client is progressing toward expected outcomes and goal achievement.

Characteristics of Evaluation

The evaluation phase and the assessment phase are similar in that they are both ongoing. When the client enters the health care continuum, initial assessment data are collected to establish a baseline. Assessment, reassessment, and evaluation continue as *long as care is provided.* Client response is compared with behaviors stated in the goal or expected outcomes, for example, reversal of symptoms, improved energy level, proper use of equipment, or

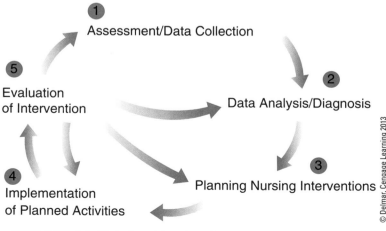

FIGURE 6:1 Relationship of evaluation to nursing process.

reduced pain. Evaluation focuses on the relationship between the care provided and the client's progress toward goal attainment.

Evaluation is not an end to the nursing process but a mechanism that ensures quality interventions. This phase helps determine if the documented plan is working and if more might be accomplished. The nurse judges the success of the previous steps of the nursing process and examines the client's response to interventions and medical treatment or therapies. Evaluation aids in analysis of the quality of nursing care provided at an institution or agency and helps determine if referral to other resources, consultation, or collaboration may be necessary. The nurse must be sensitive to subtle or obvious changes in the client's physiological condition, emotional status, and behavior. Positive and negative factors are identified, which affect the client's response. Inquiries helpful in evaluating the application of the nursing process include:

- Was assessment thorough and accurate?
- Were nursing diagnoses relevant?
- Did the client and family participate in priority problem identification and goal setting?
- Were goals specific, measurable, and realistic?
- Were expected outcomes achieved?
- Did nursing interventions and actions appropriately address the client's problems?
- Is the plan of care appropriate and accurate?
- Should any portion of the plan be modified or terminated?

Data from the above inquiry are analyzed to determine whether behaviors indicate progress toward goal achievement.

When documented, evaluation is stated in present or past tense. Refer to Table 6:1 for an example of how evaluation is documented in a care plan.

TABLE 6:1 Documenting evaluation of the care plan.

Nursing Diagnosis	Goal Statement	Nursing Interventions	Scientific Rationale	Evaluation
Parenting, Altered Related to (R/T): lack of knowledge about child development As evidenced by (AEB): statements of inability to meet child's needs, role inadequacy, frustration	Client will report comfort with role expectations within 1 week.	Assist with identifying deficits or alterations in parenting skills.	Counseling involves a mutual exchange of ideas and provides a basis for problem solving.	Client reports that he is more comfortable in role expectations.

REFLECTION EVALUATING

Evaluation, similar to assessment, is a continuous process and an essential part of professional nursing. Evaluating involves determining whether client goals and expected outcomes have been met, have been only partially met, or have not been met.

Refer back to the reflection section on implementing and the 83-year-old patient with impaired swallowing. The goal for the client was that he not experience aspiration during his hospitalization. Nursing interventions were carried out and important assessments were made by the nurse before, during, and after each intervention; then the client's response was documented. This information should be communicated to other nurses who are involved in the client's care. Evaluating is:

- Determining the client's progress or lack of progress toward achievement of expected outcomes
- Determining the effectiveness of nursing care as interventions are carried out
- Determining overall quality of care provided

The client with impaired swallowing responded favorably to nursing interventions. In this scenario, the goal is being met; therefore, planned interventions are appropriate and will most likely promote goal achievement.

Evaluating is not only determining goal achievement but is also an important process methodically used to judge:

- The value of nursing interventions
- The client's status
- The need to modify or revise the plan of care, if the goal and expected outcomes are not being met

Recall that outcome evaluation compares the client's current status with the goal and expected outcomes criteria. This process also examines all direct care activities that affect the client's status.

Review of Goals and Expected Outcomes

A **goal** is the overall desired change in the client's health status or behavior. Goals are phrased in general terms. **Expected outcomes** are stated in more specific terms. Both are directed toward the same destination. Expected outcomes may be thought of as more manageable targets advancing the client toward goal attainment. Goals and expected outcomes express behaviors to be accomplished within a specified time frame. After the behavior has been demonstrated, advancement toward problem resolution is indicated. As hospital stays become shorter, many clients are discharged before all goals are met.

Care Plan Modification

As the client responds to treatment, therapies, and nursing interventions, a change in the care plan may be warranted. Critical thought questions are asked:

- Has the expected outcome occurred?
- Is the client progressing as expected?
- Has there been a change in the client's condition?
- Is the client's health status improving?

Progress toward goal attainment most likely indicates that appropriate interventions were planned and instituted. In this case, the plan of care continues as recorded, and the client will continue to be monitored. Revisions (rewriting or amending) or modifications to the care plan are expected, however, as the client progresses to a higher level of wellness. The care plan is revised or updated to reflect the client's changing needs.

Lack of progress toward goal attainment may indicate the care plan needs modification as well. Unmet and partially met goals reactivate the nursing process sequence as previously discussed. **Modifications** to the care plan are made when needed.

Finally, when goals or desired outcomes are determined as *having been achieved* and the client no longer requires nursing assistance in this area, the nurse discontinues that portion of the care plan. Nurses continue to reassess the client for possible return of symptoms. For example, if the nursing diagnosis *Constipation* were resolved and no longer a valid concern to the client, the nurse would continue to assess function of the gastrointestinal tract.

Care Plan Evaluation and Discharge Summary

Length of stay in acute care settings continues to decrease. Preparation for discharge begins at the time of admission. The client's condition and expected outcomes dictate the type of planning required. Some agencies employ personnel with the primary responsibility of discharge planning for the client. The nurse who is caring for the individual client is responsible for ensuring that all appropriate interventions have been implemented before discharge. Additional services or facilities involved in ongoing health care include rehabilitation facilities, home health care, nursing home care, or health care clinics.

Ideally, when preparing the client for discharge, it is appropriate to evaluate the status of each nursing diagnosis prior to discharge. An evaluative statement is written, identifying the client's partial progress toward goal achievement and problem resolution. The care plan is revised for home and follow-up care. This plan is summarized in discharge instructions and documented. Additional assessment and documentation criteria may be required according to the policy and procedures of individual facilities.

KEY CONCEPTS

- Evaluation is the fifth step of the nursing process. Although it is the final step, evaluation is interwoven throughout the entire nursing process sequence. Evaluation is continuous and cyclic in nature.

- The purpose of evaluation is to judge the effectiveness of chosen interventions, nursing care, and the quality of care provided.
- As evaluation takes place, assessment of the client continues. Evaluation of goal attainment compares the client's behavior or response to the behavior or response specified in the stated goal. It is this behavior and stated time frame that make goals measurable.
- Degrees of goal attainment include the goal was met, partially met, or not met.
- As the client progresses toward a higher level of wellness, revisions or modifications to the care plan are expected. When specific problems have been resolved and no longer require intervention from the nurse, this portion of the care plan may be discontinued. Evaluation in the previously problematic area continues for possible return of signs or symptoms.

STUDENT PRACTICE: EVALUATION

Instructions

Answer the following questions:

1. What three essential cognitive skills are practiced in all steps of the nursing process? Define each skill.

   A. _____

   _____

   _____

   B. _____

   _____

   _____

   _____

   C. _____

   _____

   _____

   _____

2. Give one example of how the nurse may employ critical thinking in the following vignette: As the nurse entered the client's room, the client was holding her midchest or sternum area. The client was breathing faster than usual.

   _____

   _____

   _____

   _____

_____

_____

_____

_____

3. What is the difference between assessment and evaluation?

_____

_____

_____

_____

_____

_____

_____

4. What are the similarities between assessment and evaluation?

_____

_____

_____

_____

_____

_____

_____

5. How is evaluation documented on the care plan?

_____

_____

_____

_____

_____

_____

_____

6. What is the purpose of evaluation?

_____

_____

_____

_____

_____

_____

_____

7. What does goal attainment mean in relation to evaluation and the nursing process?

_____

_____

_____

_____

_____

_____

_____

8. When is the care plan or portions of the care plan revised, modified, or discontinued?

_____

_____

_____

_____

_____

_____

_____

_____

_____

CHAPTER 7

PUTTING IT ALL TOGETHER!

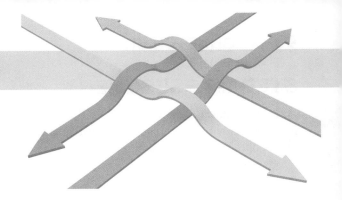

APPLICATION OF THE NURSING PROCESS

The nursing process is a cyclic, ongoing method of providing client-centered care. It is a tool used by nurses to promote organization and utilization of the steps to achieve desired outcomes, that is, goal attainment and problem resolution.

As the client enters the health care system, nurses are involved in decision making. Care is planned for the client based on data continuously collected and analyzed. Initial data collected become the database used for comparison of future data.

Nurses use skills vital to all steps of the nursing process: critical thinking, problem solving, and decision making. Critical thinking is a purposeful thought process in which deliberate questions are asked in search of meaning of data. Nurses solve problems by analyzing collected data in order to understand and make decisions regarding client needs. Decisions are made based on the nurse's understanding of scientifically based theories and knowledge of standards. These skills and others are employed as nurses interact with clients. Each interaction is an opportunity for the nurse to assess and evaluate client responses to care and medical treatment, as well as the effectiveness of care.

This chapter presents a review discussion of the nursing process. The nursing process steps are applied to a sample scenario, as if providing care to a client. A final care plan appears at the end of the chapter (Figure 7:1).

STEP 1: ASSESSMENT

Assessment includes collection, validation, organization, and interpretation of data. Initial data gathered during an interview, physical assessment, and review of diagnostic studies become the client database. These data may be used for comparison as additional data are collected. After the client enters the health care system, other sources of data may include nursing records, medical records, verbal and written consultations, relevant literature regarding the client's illness, standards indicating normal functioning against which the client is compared, and other members of the health care team working with the client. Assessment is a continuous process of collecting data to identify needs of the client and perpetuates as long as there is a need for health care.

Two categories of data are collected, subjective and objective. *Subjective* data include statements made by the client, such as feelings, perceptions, or concerns. *Objective* data include signs that are observable, measurable, or felt by someone other than the person experiencing them. Each category complements and clarifies the other.

Collected assessment data are recorded using various tools designed for that purpose. Tools should consider all aspects of the client, including physical, emotional, social, spiritual, and economic well-being.

As data are collected, verified, and validated for accuracy, the nurse assigns meaning and groups data into clusters. Data clustering is used to determine the relatedness of facts, to find patterns, and to determine if further data are needed. Related subjective and objective data are clustered together supporting the fact that a health problem exists that requires intervention.

Client Scenario

General Information

Name: Mrs. L. N.
Age: 78 years   **Gender:** Female   **Race/Ethnicity:** African American
Admitting Medical Diagnosis: Bronchitis
Admitting Weight/Height/Vital Signs: Weight, 122 pounds; height, 60 inches; blood pressure, 148/74 mm Hg; pulse, 116 beats/min; temperature, 102.0°F; respiratory rate, 26 breaths/min
Perception of Reason for Admission: Chest discomfort, dyspnea, cough, fatigue, fever
Allergies: No known food or drug allergies
Current Medications: No prescription medications; takes acetaminophen for headaches

Assessment Data

Neuro/Orientation: Answers all questions appropriately; alert, oriented to person, time, place. No sensory deficits.
Oxygenation: Reports progressive difficulty breathing over past 2 days; oxygen is being administered via nasal cannula at 2 L/min; states she is a non-smoker, however, her husband has smoked cigarettes for over 20 years; breath sounds with crackles in bilateral lower lobes; inspiratory and expiratory wheezing to bilateral mid and lower lungs; ineffective, nonproductive cough; increased use of accessory muscles; apical pulse, 116 beats/min, regular; peripheral pulses equal, regular, strong bilaterally; skin color with pale pink-yellow undertones; capillary refill sluggish, greater than 2 seconds; oxygen saturation is low; reports chest discomfort that increases with deep inhalation and cough. Mrs. N. is restless and has difficulty vocalizing.

Temperature: 102.2°F; reports elevated temperature and chills for previous 3 days.
Nutritional/Fluid: Denies difficulty chewing or swallowing food, normal appetite; has maintained oral fluid intake; no nausea or vomiting; skin is elastic with instant recoil.
Elimination: Voids without difficulty five to seven times daily; reports normal bowel pattern.
Rest/Sleep: usually retires around 9:00 p.m. and sleeps until 5:00 a.m.; however, is experiencing increased fatigue; does not feel rested after full nights sleep; no energy.
Pain Avoidance: Reports chest discomfort when she coughs or inhales deeply. Unable to rate discomfort or describe; mild headache; muscle aches.
Activity: States she usually bowls twice weekly with her husband and previously was able to perform all activities of daily living (ADLs) without difficulty; however, since becoming ill, experiences exhaustion and becomes short of breath with physical exertion. Observed dyspnea with exertion while transferring from wheelchair to bed.
Additional Data: Denies visual and hearing problems; pupils equal and reactive to light; skin is intact. Saline lock is in her right hand, and sight is without erythema or edema.
Laboratory/Diagnostic Reports: Chest radiograph reveals an acute infiltrate in left lower lung field; routine laboratory tests, including CBC, serum electrolytes, renal function and arterial blood gases, have been drawn with results pending.

This scenario represents initial assessment data collected from the client's interview and physical assessment. The nurse utilizes a data collection format approved for his or her facility. As the nurse collects data, questions are asked to verify or validate data when necessary. The nurse is now ready to organize the data, first by separating abnormal objective data (measurements and observations) from subjective data (statements and feelings that only the client can identify). Finally, the nurse clusters data to determine their relatedness and confirm that health problems or risk problems exist.

Subjective and Objective Data

Subjective Data

- Progressive difficulty breathing
- Report of elevated temperature and chills
- Chest discomfort with cough or inhalation
- Headache, muscle aches
- Fatigue
- Husband smokes (environmental exposure)
- No energy, not rested
- Dyspnea with exertion

Objective Data

- Blood pressure, 148/74 mm Hg
- Pulse, 116 beats/min
- Temperature, 102.2°F
- Respiratory rate, 26 breaths/min with use of accessory muscles
- Oxygen via nasal cannula
- Crackles to bilateral lower lobes; wheezing in bilateral lobes
- Consolidation in left lower lobe with radiograph revealing infiltrate
- Ineffective nonproductive cough
- Capillary refill sluggish
- Oxygen saturation low on room air
- Restless
- Difficulty vocalizing
- Observed dyspnea with exertion

Clustering Data (Listing problems and grouping)

Activity	Respiratory	Physical Regulation
• Fatigue; does not feel rested after sleeping • Muscle aches • Chest discomfort with cough and inhalation • Dyspnea with exertion • Restlessness	• Difficulty in breathing • Ineffective nonproductive cough • Respiratory rate increased, use of accessory muscles to breathe • Oxygen saturation low on room air, need of supplemental oxygen • Radiograph revealing infiltrate, consolidation in left lower lung, crackles auscultated in bilateral lower lobes; wheezing in bilateral lobes • Second-hand smoke exposure • Difficulty vocalizing • Restlessness	• Elevated temperature, chills • Pulse, 116 beats/min • Elevated blood pressure • Dyspnea with exertion • Increased respiratory rate • Headache

As you can see, objective and subjective data complement and clarify each other. After data are clustered, it becomes evident that health problems and risk problems exist. The care plan will be developed from initial and ongoing data collection.

STEP 2: DIAGNOSIS

Diagnosis involves critical thought and judgment to analyze, organize, and interpret assessment data. Problems, risk problems, and strengths are identified and labeled with NANDA nursing diagnoses. After labeling, the nursing diagnosis communicates specific health care needs about the client to other members of the health care team involved in care.

The data collection tool used in the scenario provides information pertaining to specific areas of functioning: comfort, respiratory function, and regulatory function. Review the list of clustered data under each category where actual problems are discovered during the assessment step. Information should be analyzed, interpreted, and labeled with nursing diagnoses.

The following is a list of actual or risk nursing diagnoses, related to (R/T) risk factors, and defining characteristics, which will be included in the care plan. Locate each nursing diagnosis in Appendix A and read the definition. Does the definition apply to Mrs. N.?

• *Gas Exchange, Impaired*
  R/T: ventilation perfusion imbalance
  As evidenced by (AEB): tachycardia, hypoxia, dyspnea, abnormal rate and depth of breathing

- *Activity Intolerance* (Level III)
  R/T: imbalance between oxygen supply and demand
  AEB: report of increasing fatigue and exhaustion, dyspnea with exertion, increased heart rate, respiratory rate, and blood pressure

Impaired Gas Exchange and *Activity Intolerance* are priority nursing diagnoses labeling *actual* client health problems. The client is exhibiting signs and symptoms in response to her medical condition. The client may be *at risk* for additional problems if her condition worsens.

STEP 3: PLANNING AND OUTCOME IDENTIFICATION

Planning the care for the client involves several steps:

- Identifying priority problems
- Setting realistic goals and expected outcomes
- Determining nursing interventions and scientific rationale
- Communicating and documenting the care plan

The planning step should involve discussing the plan with the client for input and collaboration. This encourages client participation and promotes the client's sense of control. Careful, effective planning advocates and ensures delivery of quality care.

Determining priorities involves analyzing data to discover situations requiring immediate attention. The client often communicates this during the interview or assessment. Consider Maslow's hierarchy of needs. The basic physiological needs include oxygenation, nutrition, hydration, elimination, body temperature maintenance, and pain avoidance.

In our scenario, Mrs. N. demonstrated outstanding signs and symptoms in areas of pain avoidance, oxygenation, and activity. After collaboration, she confirmed her respiratory status as the priority problem at the moment.

Establishing goals and expected outcomes follow priority problem identification. *One* overall goal is determined for each nursing diagnosis. Goals are guidelines that help to individualize nursing interventions. Goals give direction to the care plan and focus on the etiology of the problem. *Goals* are general statements indicating the intent or desired change in the client's health status, function, or behavior. *Expected outcomes* are stated in specific terms, describing methods through which the goal will be achieved.

Required components of goals include the subject (client), behavior, criteria of performance, and time frame. An optional component is the condition, referring to the aid that facilitates the performance. Goals and expected outcomes must be realistic. Review the following goals/expected outcomes for Mrs. N. *Can you identify each component of the goal statement?*

Nursing diagnosis: Gas Exchange, Impaired. R/T: ventilation perfusion imbalance. AEB: tachycardia, hypoxia, dyspnea, abnormal rate and depth of breathing.

Goal/client outcomes: Mrs. N. will demonstrate improved ventilation and absence of symptoms of respiratory distress within 24 hours.

Nursing diagnosis: Activity Intolerance (Level III). R/T: imbalance between oxygen supply and demand. AEB: report of increasing fatigue and exhaustion, dyspnea with exertion, increased heart rate, respiratory rate, and blood pressure.

Goal/client outcomes: Mrs. N. will report improved ability to perform activities without experiencing dyspnea within 48 hours after initiation of medical/nursing treatment.

Planning Nursing Interventions

Nursing interventions are activities planned and executed by the nursing team that benefit the client in a predictable manner. Interventions are selected based on scientific principles and knowledge of behavioral and physical sciences. Nurses use deliberate thought, decision making, and problem solving to determine actions that will aid in elimination, prevention, or reduction of the cause of the problem or nursing diagnosis. Nursing interventions are developed from the etiology of each nursing diagnosis. Generally, several interventions should be identified for each goal.

Interventions are selected based on the nurse's understanding of scientific principle and psychosocial or developmental theories. Understanding of the human body and mind allows for certain expected responses when interventions are carried out. The term *scientific rationale* is the underlying reason for choosing a specific intervention. *Do you remember?*

Explain the process of locating scientific rationales.

_____

_____

_____

Can you list four or more sources?

_____

_____

_____

Describe steps taken when locating scientific rationale.

_____

_____

_____

Nursing interventions and scientific rationale for our scenario follow:

Nursing diagnosis: Gas Exchange, Impaired. R/T: ventilation perfusion imbalance. AEB: tachycardia, hypoxia, dyspnea, abnormal rate and depth of breathing.

Goal/client outcomes: Mrs. N. will demonstrate improved ventilation and absence of symptoms of respiratory distress within 24 hours.

Nursing interventions and *scientific rationales*:

1. Maintain elevated head of bed. *Promotes optimal chest expansion and drainage of secretions.*
2. Encourage and maintain adequate fluid intake. *Helps to mobilize lung secretions and improve expectoration.*
3. Administer prescribed medications, such as antibiotics. *To treat underlying condition and improve respiratory status.*
4. Encourage adequate rest and promote calm environment. *Helps limit oxygen needs/consumption.*

Nursing diagnosis: Activity Intolerance (Level III). R/T: imbalance between oxygen supply and demand. AEB: report of increasing fatigue and exhaustion, dyspnea with exertion, increased heart rate, respiratory rate, and blood pressure.

Goal/client outcomes: Mrs. N. will report improved ability to perform activities without experiencing dyspnea within 48 hours after initiation of medical/nursing treatment.

Nursing interventions and *scientific rationales*:

1. Evaluate current limitations as compared to usual activity status. *Provides a comparative baseline.*
2. Provide adequate rest periods between activities. *To limit fatigue and to prevent overexertion.*
3. Assist with activities and encourage patient to increase activity levels gradually. *Conserves and improves energy level.*

After the plan of care is developed it is shared with other members of the health care team involved in caring for the client. The plan is communicated verbally and through written documentation. The care plan records health care needs, coordinates nursing care, promotes continuity of care, encourages communication within the health care team, and promotes quality nursing care.

STEP 4: IMPLEMENTATION

During implementation, planned nursing interventions are executed. This step begins with assessment and evaluation of the client prior to initiating care. Each interaction with the client is an opportunity to assess, collect ongoing data, and compare data with the client's baseline. Nurses apply scientific knowledge and understanding, analytical skills, and deliberate thought to interpret ongoing data collection. Priority interventions are carried out first. However, nurses may perform interventions for more than one problem at the same time.

The nurse is legally required to record all interventions implemented as well as observations related to the client's response to treatments. Written documentation provides a legal record and can be reviewed by other health care team members involved in the patient's care.

STEP 5: EVALUATION

The *evaluation* phase measures the effectiveness of nursing care and the quality of care provided. However, evaluation, like assessment, is not a static activity but is ongoing and cyclic, never ceasing. As interventions are carried out, client *responses* are evaluated, and the client is reassessed.

Questions are asked about the appropriateness and effectiveness of the intervention and the client's response to medical treatment, therapies, and nursing interventions. Are goals being met? If not, answers are sought to determine why.

Evaluation of the care plan focuses on changes in the client's health status, that is, if the client is progressing toward goal attainment. As the client's health status changes, the care plan is revised to reflect the changing needs.

Lack of progress toward goal attainment may indicate that the care plan needs revisions or modifications. The nursing process sequence is reactivated and assessment begins again. Again, collected data are analyzed, organized, and interpreted. All planning is compared to that previously determined, searching for omissions or inaccuracies. A revised care plan is developed and executed.

During evaluation, when goals and expected outcomes are determined as having been achieved and the client no longer requires nursing assistance in this area, this portion of the care plan is discontinued. Nurses will continue to assess and evaluate the client for possible return of symptoms.

The completed care plan for Mrs. N is provided in Figure 7:1.

STUDENT PRACTICE

Instructions

Read the case scenario and apply the five steps of the nursing process. Identify three appropriate nursing diagnoses (with *R/T* and *AEB* or *risk factors*). For each nursing diagnosis, provide one goal/expected outcome, three nursing interventions with scientific rationale, and one evaluative statement. The care plan form is attached.

General Information

Name: Mr. Stephen (Tipper) Carlson
Age: 45 years   **Gender:** Male   **Race/Ethnicity:** Caucasian
Admitting Medical Diagnosis: S/P Motor vehicle accident (MVA) with fractured pelvis and multiple contusions
Admitting Weight/Height/Vital Signs: Weight, 165 pounds; height, 67 inches; temperature, 99.0°F; blood pressure, 144/88 mm Hg; heart rate, 90 beats/min; respiratory rate, 22 breaths/min.
Client's Perception of Reason for Admission: "I was in a car accident."
Allergies: None
Current Medications: No prescription medications; no over-the-counter (OTC) medications.
Past Medical History: Appendectomy at age 8 years.

Assessment Data

Neuro/Orientation: Alert, oriented to person, time, place.
Cardiovascular: Denies dyspnea; states he is a nonsmoker; breath sounds clear to auscultation bilaterally; no cough; apical pulse, 90 beats/min and regular; peripheral pulses equal, regular, and strong bilaterally; skin warm, pink, and dry; capillary refill less than 2 seconds.

Nursing Diagnosis	Goal/Expected Outcomes	Nursing Interventions	Scientific Rationale	Evaluation
Gas Exchange, Impaired R/T: ventilation perfusion imbalance AEB: tachycardia, hypoxia, dyspnea, abnormal rate and depth of breathing	Mrs. N. will demonstrate improved ventilation and absence of symptoms of respiratory distress within 24 hours. Note: each required component is included in this goal statement	1. Maintain elevated head of bed at all times. 2. Encourage and maintain adequate fluid intake. 3. Administer prescribed medications, such as antibiotics. 4. Encourage adequate rest and promote calm environment.	1. Promotes optimal chest expansion and drainage of secretions. 2. Helps to mobilize lung secretions and improve expectoration of secretions. 3. To treat underlying condition and improve respiratory status. 4. Helps limit oxygen needs/consumption.	Pulse oximeter, reading 98% oxygen saturation throughout shift. Respiratory rate, 20 breaths/min. Mrs. N. denies shortness of breath. Note: evaluation is reported in present or past tense.
Activity Intolerance (Level III) R/T: imbalance between oxygen supply and demand AEB: report of increasing fatigue and exhaustion, dyspnea with exertion, increased heart rate, respiratory rate, and blood pressure	Mrs. N. will report improved ability to perform activities without experiencing dyspnea within 48 hours after initiation of medical/nursing treatment.	1. Evaluate current limitations compared with usual activity status. 2. Provide adequate rest periods between activities. 3. Assist with activities and encourage patient to increase activity levels gradually.	1. Provides a comparative baseline. 2. To limit fatigue and to prevent overexertion. 3. Conserves and improves energy level. Note: each nursing intervention requires scientific rationale	Mrs. N. is able to assist in self-care without becoming short of breath.

FIGURE 7:1 Documented care plan for Mrs. N.

Nutritional/ Fluid: Denies difficulty chewing or swallowing food; normal appetite; no nausea or vomiting; skin is elastic with instant recoil; prescribed nothing by mouth (NPO) at this time.

Elimination: Foley catheter to gravity drainage with clear, light yellow urine; reports usually bowel elimination pattern as once each day but has had no bowel movement for 4 days; abdominal bowel sounds are hypoactive in all four quadrants.

Rest/Sleep: Usually retires around 10:00 p.m. and sleeps until 5:00 a.m.

Pain Avoidance: Reports severe pain to pelvic area, rated as "7" on a scale of 0 to 10, described as "intense, ripping sensation with muscle spasms"; muscle aches throughout body.

Activity: Previously active, no deficits. At this time, physician prescribed complete bed rest with continuous pelvic traction.

Additional Data: No visual or hearing deficits; pupils equal and reactive to light; superficial wounds noted to left, lateral forearm, wrist, and hand with no erythema, no edema. Ecchymosis (bruising) observed to left, lateral pelvic and abdominal regions. Abdomen is soft with mild tenderness to left upper and lower abdomen when lightly palpated.

Laboratory/Diagnostic Reports: Computed tomography (CT) reveals fractured left pelvis. Laboratory findings are unremarkable.

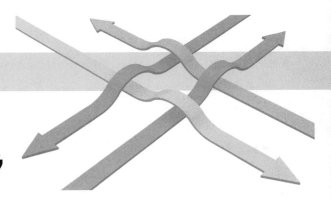

CHAPTER 8

CLIENT-CENTERED CONCEPT MAPPING

Upon completion of this chapter, the student should be able to:

▶ Identify the purpose of client-centered concept mapping utilizing the nursing process.

▶ Correlate critical thinking as it relates to the nursing process and client-centered concept mapping.

▶ Describe how client-centered concept mapping complements the nursing process.

CONCEPT MAPPING

Concept mapping, or mind mapping, has been around for several years. It is viewed as a method of promoting critical thinking in nursing education. Concept maps may be developed from a single topic or focus, such as a pathological condition or disease process, for the purpose of understanding that condition. In addition, concept maps may be created as a method of study by mapping out pathophysiological processes of one or more health care conditions and presented in combination with the nursing process. Many nursing students are better able to visualize how one condition affects another and how the client responds to implemented medical or nursing interventions. In practice, concept mapping can be used in the clinical setting as a method to develop and maintain the client's plan of care.

Concept mapping, similar to the nursing process, is a nonlinear means used to collect data, interpret, plan, analyze, and evaluate client care. This chapter will explain and demonstrate how to develop a client-centered concept map using the five-step nursing process as discussed in previous chapters. Examples and activities provide an interactive approach to concept mapping throughout each phase of the nursing process. For this purpose, the sample client scenario relating to Mrs. N. from Chapter 7 will be utilized.

APPLICATION OF CONCEPT MAPPING

The nursing process is the foundation of providing client-centered care. Recall that the nursing process consists of five steps: assessment, diagnosis, planning, implementation, and evaluation. The five steps of the nursing process will be further broken down into critical thinking and interactive exercises.

GETTING STARTED

The first step of developing a client-centered concept map involves data collection. Review the clinical record to identify current health problems, past medical history (PMH), medication record, laboratory and diagnostic test results, physical assessment data, current treatments ordered, and any other data pertaining to the client's care. Perform a complete physical assessment on the client to gather current clinical findings. The nurse or nursing student now has the necessary information to begin building a working concept map.

The central "figure" of the concept map represents the client and the reason for seeking medical attention or the chief complaint. Additional information to include will be the client's PMH, allergies, and any other essential information for the client's admission (Figure 8:1). Remember to follow HIPAA guidelines when using client data in the clinical setting.

Depending on the client's current and past medical condition(s), data may range anywhere from simple to complex. Begin the concept map by branching off of the central figure with each health care condition or medical diagnosis (current reason for hospitalization). Include the appropriate PMH and risk factors (modifiable and nonmodifiable). It is beneficial to identify and briefly explain the pathophysiology of each health related condition. Completing this step will help increase the understanding of the disease process and the connection or linkages among assessment findings, PMH, medical and nursing interventions, laboratory and diagnostic findings, and pharmacologic treatment.

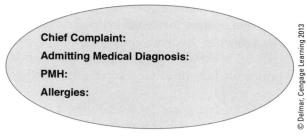

Chief Complaint:

Admitting Medical Diagnosis:

PMH:

Allergies:

© Delmar, Cengage Learning 2013

FIGURE 8:1 Client-Specific Data.

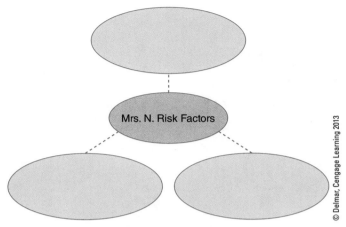

© Delmar, Cengage Learning 2013

FIGURE 8:2 Risk Factors.

STUDENT INTERACTIVE ACTIVITY

Review the scenario found in Chapter 7 for Mrs. N. Using the nursing diagnosis handbook or a medical-surgical textbook, identify all risk factors associated with bronchitis. Add the risk factors that pertain to Mrs. N onto the concept map (Figure 8:2).

ASSESSMENT

Based on data collected during the assessment phase, the client-centered concept map can now be developed. Consider the client-specific data documented in Figure 8:1 (chief complaint, admitting medical diagnosis, PMH, and allergies). Also consider and review physical assessment data. Identify all signs and symptoms associated with the medical diagnosis.

STUDENT INTERACTIVE ACTIVITY

Concept Mapping: Assessment

Mrs. N was admitted with bronchitis. Review bronchitis in the nursing medical-surgical or pathophysiology textbook. Branching off of Figure 8:3, add *expected* signs and symptoms (S/S) of bronchitis found in the resource to the concept map.

Next, review client-specific data from the sample scenario assessment, including the signs and symptoms Mrs. N is exhibiting. For example, if *fever* was one expected sign or symptom for bronchitis listed in the medical-surgical textbook, the nursing student would draw a shape linking fever with Mrs. N's assessment temperature measured as 102.2°F. Using Figure 8:4, fill in the client-specific assessment data.

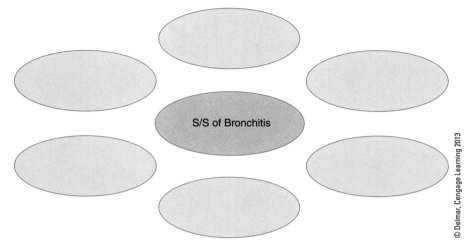

FIGURE 8:3 Bronchitis Signs and Symptoms.

© Delmar, Cengage Learning 2013

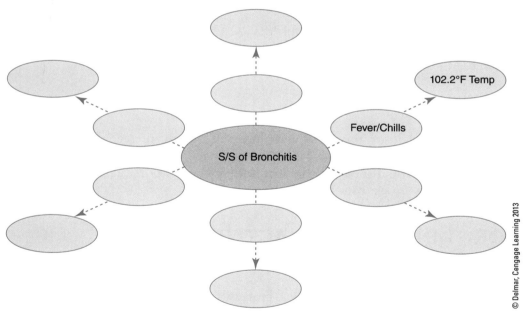

FIGURE 8:4 Client Signs and Symptoms of Bronchitis.

© Delmar, Cengage Learning 2013

NURSING DIAGNOSIS

In this step, the nursing student should analyze, organize, and interpret assessment data and then identify actual and risk nursing diagnoses from the problem list that has been created. Chapters 2 and 3 explain how to analyze, organize, and interpret assessment data; create a problem list from collected data; and correctly label actual or risk problems using NANDA Nursing Diagnoses. Review these chapters as needed.

STUDENT INTERACTIVE ACTIVITY

Using Figure 8:5, enter problems identified from Mrs. N's case scenario. Notice that Mrs. N is at the center of this entry. The problem list will be further broken down into the top three NANDA nursing diagnoses.

Refer to Figure 8:5 and identify priority problems. In Mrs. N's scenario, the admitting medical diagnosis is bronchitis, she has no PMH, and the only known risk factor is environmental exposure from second-hand smoke.

STUDENT INTERACTIVE ACTIVITY

Using Figures 8:6 to 8:8, formulate and add the top three NANDA nursing diagnoses.

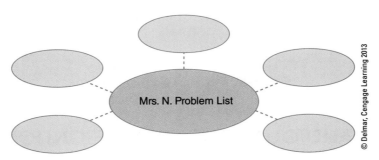

FIGURE 8:5 Client Problem List.

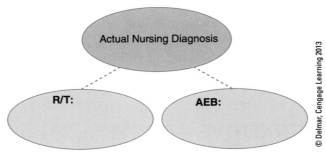

FIGURE 8:6 Nursing Diagnosis 1.

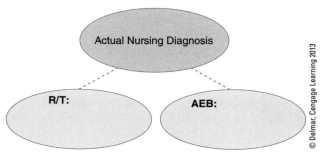

FIGURE 8:7 Nursing Diagnosis 2.

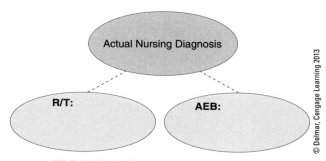

FIGURE 8:8 Nursing Diagnosis 3.

PLANNING AND OUTCOME IDENTIFICATION

Next, identify the client's goals and expected outcomes. Remember that goals and expected outcomes should be specific to the client, measurable, attainable, content specific, and time specific. Refer to Figure 8:9 as goals or expected outcomes are formulated to ensure that they are structured correctly. Review Chapter 4, "Planning," for additional information on writing goals and expected outcomes and additional steps involved in the planning phase.

After the goals and expected outcomes have been identified, nursing interventions are selected that will promote goal attainment and ultimately problem resolution. Nursing interventions are selected based on scientific principles and knowledge of behavioral and physical sciences. Nursing interventions are then planned and performed by the nursing team.

STUDENT INTERACTIVE ACTIVITY

Write one goal or expected outcome for each of the three nursing diagnoses identified in Figures 8:10 to 8:12. Use the etiology or cause of the problem that is provided to help guide development of each goal.

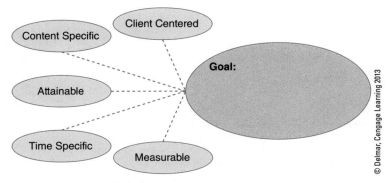

FIGURE 8:9 Goal or Expected Outcome.

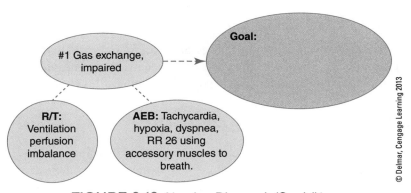

FIGURE 8:10 Nursing Diagnosis/Goal #1.

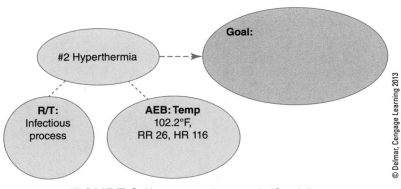

FIGURE 8:11 Nursing Diagnosis/Goal #2.

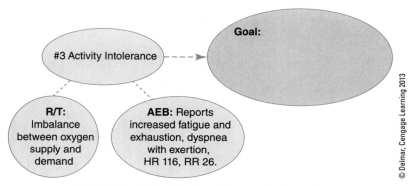

FIGURE 8:12 Nursing Diagnosis/Goal #3.

STUDENT INTERACTIVE ACTIVITY

As a self-check, compare *your* goals from figures 8:10, 8:11, and 8:12 with the goals provided in Figures 8:13, 8:14, and 8:15. Make sure the goals and expected outcomes meet the criteria of being attainable, measurable, content specific, time specific, and client directed.

CONCEPT MAPPING EXERCISE

Using Figures 8:13 to 8:15, break down each goal. For example, in Figure 8:13, the goal is *Demonstrate improved ventilation and absence of respiratory symptoms of respiratory distress within 24 hours.* One of the goal identifiers is time specific. This goal would meet the time-specific criteria because the goal should be met within 24 hours. This activity ensures that each goal or expected outcome meets required criteria.

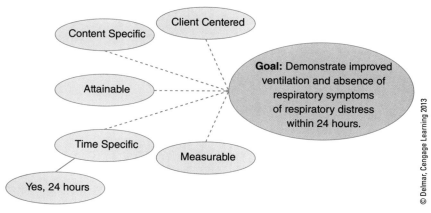

FIGURE 8:13 Client Goal 1.

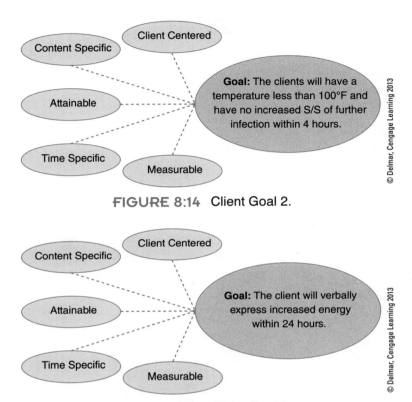

FIGURE 8:14   Client Goal 2.

FIGURE 8:15   Client Goal 3.

IMPLEMENTATION

Nursing interventions include key areas of assessment and monitoring as well as procedures or other therapeutic interventions. Therapeutic nursing interventions may involve client teaching, client and family teaching, or therapeutic communication. Throughout each clinical day, the client's assessment and effectiveness of interventions should be documented. Important information to document includes the client's status before the nursing interventions, during the interventions, and after the interventions have been carried out. Nursing interventions may change according to the needs of the client. Be prepared to identify the reason you selected a specific nursing intervention. Additional information about scientific rationales can be found in Chapter 4.

STUDENT INTERACTIVE ACTIVITY

Place a content holder for the goal in the center of the concept map for the first or highest priority nursing diagnosis. In the case scenario, *Impaired Gas Exchange* was selected as having greatest importance. Next, add each nursing intervention and scientific rationale. As nursing interventions are carried out, document the client's response to the intervention.

CONCEPT MAPPING EXERCISE

In Figure 8:16, add the nursing interventions, scientific rationales, and possible client responses in the appropriate content holders.

Practice adding appropriate data as discussed above to the Figures 8:17 and 8:18.

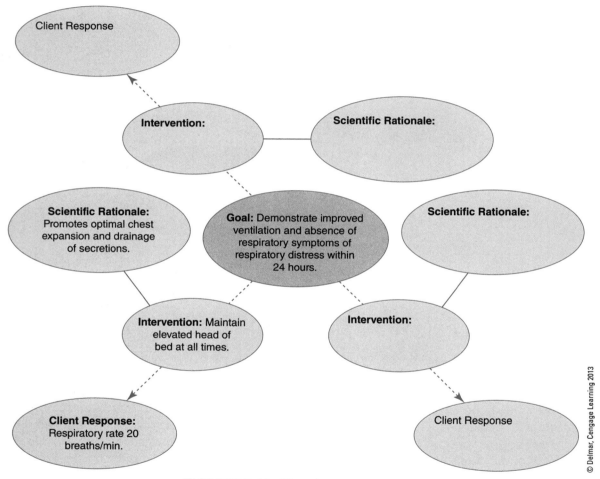

FIGURE 8:16 Client Interventions 1.

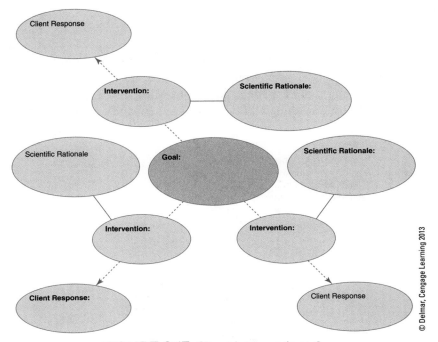

FIGURE 8:17 Client Interventions 2.

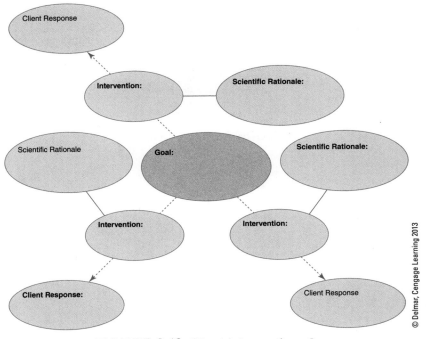

FIGURE 8:18 Client Interventions 3.

EVALUATION

The evaluation process measures whether or not the goal or expected outcome was achieved through nursing care. In Figure 8:19, the client responses to the nursing interventions are directly linked to whether or not the goal or outcome was realized. Based on the client responses to the nursing interventions and the goal identifiers, document whether the goal was met, not met, or partially met. See Figure 8:19 for an example of how to document the client's response to nursing care.

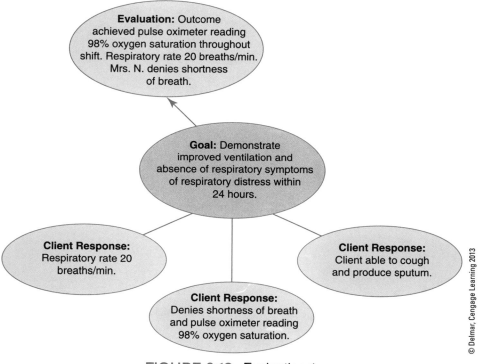

FIGURE 8:19 Evaluation 1.

CONCEPT MAPPING EXERCISE

Complete the concept map exercise found in Figures 8:20 and 8:21 based on previous activities.

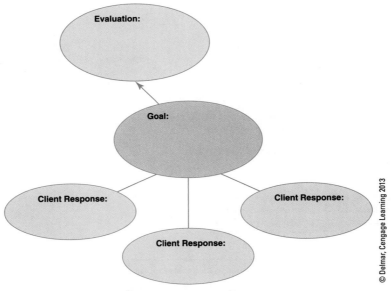

FIGURE 8:20   Evaluation 2.

PUTTING IT ALL TOGETHER

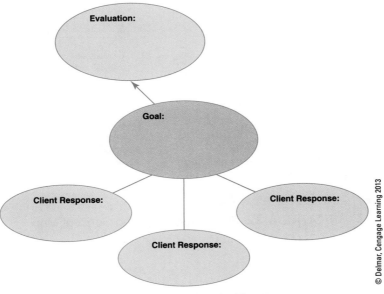

FIGURE 8:21   Evaluation 3.

CONCEPT MAPPING EXERCISE

Complete the client-centered concept map in Figure 8:22.

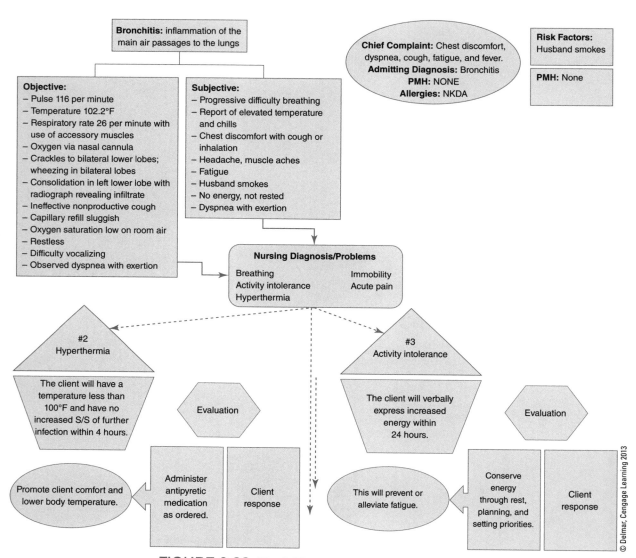

FIGURE 8:22 Final Client-centered Concept Map.

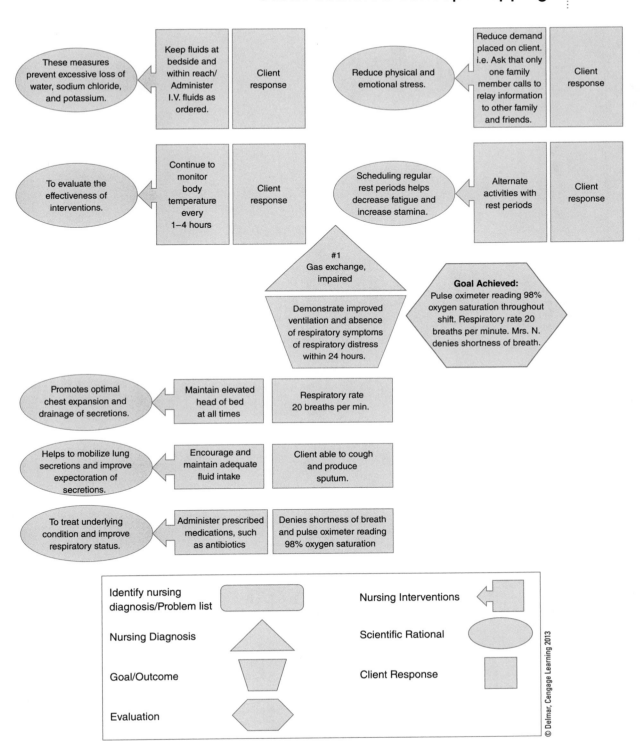

FIGURE 8:22 (*Continued*)

GLOSSARY

KEY TERMS

Actual nursing diagnosis: a label approved by NANDA, classifying specific client problems or needs

Analyze: the process of rationalizing, questioning, and classifying information to reach a conclusion about a client's needs

Assessment: the effect of gathering data, organizing the data, and then documenting the data

Auscultation: listening for sounds within the body, usually with a stethoscope

Baseline data: information initially collected, forming the client's database, used for future comparison

Care plan: written documentation of the second and third steps of the nursing process, which cites the client's problems/needs, goals/outcomes of care, and nursing interventions to treat the problems/needs

Client centered: focused on the client

Closed question: communication technique consisting of questions that can be answered briefly with yes-or-no or one-word responses

Closure: the phase of the interview in which all information has been collected and summarized

Collaboration: an act of communicating with other disciplines or parties for the purpose of decision making or problem solving

Collaborative problem: monitoring for the onset of certain physiological risk complications

Confidentiality: nondisclosure of information obtained by the health care team about a client; this information is considered privileged and cannot be disclosed to a third party without the client's consent

Critical thinking: a purposeful, deliberate method of thinking used in search for meaning

Data clustering: technique used to group related or like data; helps determine relatedness of data; provides confirmation of existing problem

Decision making: a skill used throughout the nursing process; process of applying judgments based on systematic and scientific theories

Defining characteristics: clinical criteria representing the presence of diagnostic facts; signs and symptoms indicating a specific nursing diagnosis

Dependent nursing interventions: actions requiring an order from a physician or another health care professional

Diagnosis: classification of a disease, condition, or human response determined by scientific evaluation of signs and symptoms, history, and diagnostic studies

Discharge planning: planning that requires analysis of the client's present health status and anticipates the client's needs after discharge for continued care

Discontinue: to terminate the portion of the care plan after the client has achieved the goal

Documentation: the process of recording assessment data, the client's health status, care provided, and response to care; includes written evidence of the interactions between and among health care professionals, clients and their families, and health care organizations

Etiology: cause or condition most likely to be involved in the development of a problem

Evaluation: appraisal of results through judicious reasoning; the fifth step of the nursing process

Evaluative statement: written statement identifying the client's progress toward goal achievement and problem resolution

Expected outcome: probable results; a detailed statement describing methods through which a goal will be achieved

Focus charting: a documentation method that includes written evidence of data, action, and response (DAR)

Goal: broad aim, intent, or objective

Goal attainment: achieved when the subject of the goal demonstrates the stated behavior within the specified time frame

Holistic: caring for the total person, including physical, emotional, social, spiritual, and economic needs of the client

Implementation: the fourth step of the nursing process during which nursing interventions specified in the care plan are executed

Independent nursing interventions: nursing actions initiated by the nurse, not requiring direction or an order from another health care professional

Inspection: systematic process of observation, which includes visual examination of the external surface of the body, as well as its movements and posture

Interdependent nursing interventions: nursing actions developed in collaboration or consultation with other health care professionals to gain another's viewpoint

Interpret: analyze the meaning and its significance

Interview: a communication exchange between the client and nurse

Introduction phase: the phase of an interview in which the goals of the interview are stated

The Joint Commission: formerly the Joint Commission on Accreditation of Healthcare Organizations (JCAHO): a surveying body that certifies clinical and organization performance of an institution following established guidelines

Kardex: a condensed reference tool used during change-of-shift report and as a quick reference throughout the shift; this tool includes basic client care information

Long-term goal: goal that may not be achieved prior to discharge from care but may require continued attention, usually over weeks to months

Measurable: able to be quantified

Medical diagnosis: illness, condition, or pathological state for which treatment is directed by a licensed physician

Modification: alteration or revision of original care plan

NANDA: North American Nursing Diagnosis Association, international group responsible for the development and refinement of nursing diagnoses

Narrative charting: a documentation method for which the nurse records complete data relating to the client as progress notes, sometimes supplementing notes with flow sheets

Nursing diagnosis: a label approved by NANDA identifying specific client problems/needs; means of describing health problems which nurses are licensed to treat, including physical, sociological, or psychological; the process of identifying client problems and needs; recognized as the second step of the nursing process

Nursing interventions: prescriptions for specific actions to be carried out by nurses to promote, maintain, or restore health; specified activities executed by the nursing team that benefit the client in a predictable manner

Nursing process: an orderly, step-by-step, problem-solving method of providing nursing care; the five steps are assessment, diagnosis, planning, implementation, and evaluation

Objective data: what can be observed, measured, or felt by someone other than the person experiencing the phenomenon

Observation: skill of watching thoughtfully and deliberately using the senses, touch, sight, smell, and hearing

Open-ended question: interviewing technique that promotes client elaboration about a particular concern or problem

Palpation: process of examining by applying the hands or fingers to the external surface of the body to detect evidence of disease or abnormalities in organs

Percussion: physical examination technique that uses fingertips, cup of the hand, fist, or percussion hammer to hear sounds or feel vibrations

PIE charting: a method of documentation that includes written evidence of each problem, intervention, and evaluation

Planning: the third step of the nursing process, which includes identifying priority problems and interventions, setting realistic goals and expected outcomes, determining appropriate nursing interventions and scientific rationale, determining collaboration needs, and communicating the proposed care plan through documentation

Prioritize: to impose an order or rank of precedence

Priority: estimated to be more important

Problem: the identified label of a client's health problem or response to the medical condition or therapy for which nursing may intervene; also known as the nursing diagnosis

Problem solving: the procedure of deliberate, thoughtful steps instituted for data collection, problem identification, planning for resolution, and execution of interventions

Problem statement: consists of the diagnostic label (NANDA nursing diagnosis), etiology or risk factor, and defining characteristics (if stating an actual problem)

Process: a series of planned actions or operations directed toward a particular result or goal

Rationale: the underlying reason behind a specific response

Reporting: includes verbal communication of facts regarding the client's health status and care being provided

Revision: the process of rewriting, amending, or improving

Risk nursing diagnosis: diagnostic label preceded by the phrase *risk for*; determined for potential problems the client is at risk for developing in which specific risk factors are present

Short-term goal: goal that usually must be met prior to discharge or progress to a less acute level of care; goal usually met within hours or days

Social communication: casual conversation that is spontaneous and with no planned agenda

Strength: area of positive functioning in the client, used to support the care plan, such as the desire to maintain a healthy diet, family support, or desire to get well

Subjective data: symptom; what the client reports, believes, or feels

Therapeutic communication: conversation that is purposeful, goal directed, focused on the client, and planned, creating a beneficial outcome for the client

Validation: the process of ascertaining that data are factual

Verification: process of providing confirmation or proof

Wellness diagnosis: a judgment based upon a client's transition from a specific level of health to a higher level of health

Wellness nursing diagnosis: diagnostic label preceded by the phrase *potential for enhanced*, determined when a client has indicated a desire to attain a higher level of wellness in a particular area

Working phase: the phase of the interview that focuses on data collection

BIBLIOGRAPHY

Ackley, Betty J., & Ladwig, Gail B. (2011). *Nursing diagnosis handbook: An evidence-based guide to planning care* (9th ed.). St. Louis, MO. Mosby Elsevier.

Ackley, Betty J., & Ladwig, Gail B. (2011). *Nursing diagnosis handbook: A guide to planning care* (3rd ed.). Maryland Heights, MO. Mosby Elsevier.

American Nurses Association. (2004). *Nursing: Scope and standards of practice.* Washington, DC: Author.

Benner, P. (1984). *From novice to expert.* Menlo Park, CA: Addison-Wesley Publishers.

DeLaune, Sue C., & Ladner, Patricia K. (2011). *Fundamentals of nursing: Standards and practice* (4th ed.). New York: Cengage Delmar Learning.

Clayton, L.H. (2006). Concept mapping: An effective, active teaching-learning method. *Nursing Education Perspectives* 27:4, 197–203.

Estes, M.E.Z. (2009). *Health assessment and physical examination* (4th ed.). New York: Cengage Delmar Learning.

Lippincott, Williams & Wilkins. (2009). *Chart smart: A to Z guide to better nursing documentation.* Philadelphia: LWW.

NANDA. (2009). *Nursing diagnoses: Definitions & classification 2009–2011.* Iowa: Wiley-Blackwell.

Nightingale, Florence. (1969). *Notes on nursing: What it is, and what it is not.* New York: Dover.

Seaback, Wanda W. (2006). *Nursing process: Concepts and application.* (2nd ed.). Clifton Park, NY: Cengage Delmar Learning.

University of Iowa (n.d.). *Nursing interventions classification.* Retrieved July 28, 2004, from http://www.nursing.uiowa.edu.

University of Iowa (n.d.). *Nursing outcomes classification.* Retrieved July 28, 2004, from http://www.nursing.uiowa.edu.

U.S. Department of Health and Human Services. *Health information services.* Retrieved on November 12, 2011, at http://www.hhs.gov/ocr/privacy/hipaa/understanding/index.html

Wilkinson, Judith M. (2012). *Nursing process and critical thinking* (5th ed.). Upper Saddle River, NJ. Pearson.

INDEX